Manual of Coronary Chronic Total Occlusion Interventions

Manual of Coronary Chronic Total Occlusion Interventions

A Step-by-Step Approach

Emmanouil S. Brilakis, MD, PhD

VA North Texas Health Care System and University of Texas Southwestern Medical School, Dallas, TX

AMSTERDAM • BOSTON • HEIDELBERG • LONDON
NEW YORK • OXFORD • PARIS • SAN DIEGO
SAN FRANCISCO • SINGAPORE • SYDNEY • TOKYO

Academic Press is an imprint of Elsevier

Academic Press is an imprint of Elsevier
225 Wyman Street, Waltham, MA 02451, USA
525 B Street, Suite 1800, San Diego, CA 92101-4495, USA
32 Jamestown Road, London NW1 7BY, UK

Notice

British Library Cataloguing-in-Publication Data
A catalogue record for this book is available from the British Library

Library of Congress Cataloging-in-Publication Data
Application submitted

ISBN: 978-0-12-420129-3

For information on all Academic Press publications
visit our website at store.elsevier.com

13 14 15 16 17   10 9 8 7 6 5 4 3 2 1

  Working together
to grow libraries in
developing countries

www.elsevier.com • www.bookaid.org

Dedication

To Nicole, Stelios, and Thomas

Contents

For any questions, comments, or suggestions regarding this manual please contact Emmanouil Brilakis
at esbrilakis@gmail.com

List of Contributors

Emmanouil S. Brilakis Editor, MD, PhD Director, Cardiac Catheterization Laboratories, VA North Texas Healthcare System; Associate Professor of Medicine, University of Texas Southwestern Medical School, Dallas, Texas

Tayo Addo, MD Program Director, Interventional Cardiology Fellowship Program, Assistant Professor of Medicine, University of Texas, Southwestern Medical School, Dallas, Texas

Khaldoon Alaswad, MD, FACC, FSCAI, RVT Director, Cardiovascular Catheterization Laboratory Appleton Medical Center and Theda Clark Medical Center, Appleton, Wisconsin

Subhash Banerjee, MD Chief of Cardiology, VA North Texas Healthcare System; Associate Professor of Medicine, University of Texas, Southwestern Medical School, Dallas, Texas

Christopher E. Buller, MD Director, Cardiac Catheterization & Intervention, St. Michael's Hospital; Professor of Medicine, University of Toronto, Toronto, Canada

M. Nicholas Burke, MD Minneapolis Heart Institute and Foundation, Minneapolis, Minnesota

Mauro Carlino, MD Invasive Cardiology Unit, San Raffaele Scientific Institute, Milan, Italy

Charles E. Chambers, MD Professor of Medicine and Radiology, Penn State University School of Medicine, Hershey, Pennsylvania

James W. Choi, MD, FACC, FSCAI Cardiology Consultants of Texas; Director, Interventional Cardiology Fellowship, Baylor Heart and Vascular Hospital at Baylor University Medical Center, Dallas, Texas; Associate Professor of Medicine, Texas A&M College of Medicine, Temple, Texas

Antonio Colombo, MD Director Interventional Cardiology, San Raffaele Hospital and Columbus Hospital, Milan, Italy

Stephen L. Cook, MD Director, Cardiac Catheterization Laboratory, Oregon Heart & Vascular Institute, PeaceHealth Sacred Heart Medical Center, Springfield, Oregon

Kevin J. Croce, MD, PhD Interventional Cardiology, Brigham and Women's Hospital, Harvard Medical School, Boston, Massachusetts

David V. Daniels, MD Palo Alto Medical Foundation, Palo Alto, California

Tony J. DeMartini, MD Boston Scientific Natick, Massachusetts

Amish J. Desai, MD, FACC Swedish Heart and Vascular, Seattle, Washington

Parag Doshi, MD, FACC, FSCAI President, Chicago Cardiology Institute, Schaumburg, Illinois

Javier Escaned, MD, PhD, FESC Cardiovascular Institute Hospital Clínico San Carlos, Madrid, Spain

Alfredo R. Galassi, MD, FACC, FESC, FSCAI Associate Professor of Cardiology, Postgraduate School of Cardiology, Department of Medical Sciences and Pediatrics, University of Catania; Director of the Catheterization Laboratory and Cardiovascular Interventional Unit, Cannizzaro Hospital, Catania, Italy

Santiago Garcia, MD Staff Interventional Cardiologist, Minneapolis VA Healthcare System; Assistant Professor of Medicine, University of Minnesota, Minneapolis, Minnesota

Cosmo Godino, MD Cardio-Thoracic-Vascular Department, San Raffaele Scientific Institute, Milan, Italy

Jerrold Grodin, MD Interventional Cardiologist, VA North Texas Healthcare System; Assistant Professor of Medicine, University of Texas Southwestern Medical School, Dallas, Texas

Colm Hanratty, MD, FRCPI Department of Cardiology, Belfast Health and Social Care Trust, Belfast, Northern Ireland

Elizabeth M. Holper, MD, MPH Medical City Hospital, Dallas, Texas

Farouc Jaffer, MD, PhD, FACC, FAHA Associate Professor of Medicine, Harvard Medical School; Attending Interventional Cardiologist, Massachusetts General Hospital, Boston, Massachusetts

David E. Kandzari, MD, FACC, FSCAI Director, Interventional Cardiology and Chief Scientific Officer, Piedmont Heart Institute, Atlanta, Georgia

Dimitri Karmpaliotis, MD, FACC, FSCAI Interventional Cardiology, Piedmont Heart Institute, Atlanta, Georgia

Anna Kotsia, MD Research Associate, VA North Texas Healthcare System and University of Texas UT Southwestern Medical Center, Dallas, Texas

Chad Kugler President and General Manager, Bridgrepoint Medical, Minneapolis, Minnesota

Dharam J. Kumbhani, MD, SM, MRCP, FACC Assistant Professor, Interventional Cardiology, Department of Internal Medicine, University of Texas Southwestern Medical Center, Dallas, Texas

Thierry Lefèvre, MD, FSCAI, FESC Institut Cardiovasculaire Paris Sud, Massy, France

Nicholas J. Lembo, MD, FACC, FSCAI Piedmont Heart Institute, Atlanta, Georgia

Martin B. Leon, MD Professor of Medicine, Director, Cardiac Catheterization Laboratories and Center for Interventional Vascular Therapy, Columbia University Medical Center, New York

William Lombardi, MD, FACC, FSCAI Peacehealth St. Joseph Hospital Bellingham, Washington

Michael Luna, MD Assistant Professor of Medicine, University of Texas Southwestern Medical School, Dallas, Texas

Roxana Mehran, MD Professor of Medicine, Mount Sinai School of Medicine; Director of Interventional Cardiovascular Research and Clinical Trials, Zena and Michael A. Wiener Cardiovascular Institute; Chief Scientific Officer of Clinical Trials Center, Cardiovascular Research Foundation, New York, New York

Jeffrey Moses, MD Professor of Medicine, Columbia University Medical Center, New York, New York

William J Nicholson, MD York Hospital−Interventional Cardiology, York, Pennsylvania

Göran Olivecrona, MD, PhD, FSCAI Chairman, Working Group on Interventional Cardiology, Swedish Society of Cardiology; Department of Cardiology, Skane University Hospital-Lund, Lund, Sweden

Ashish Pershad, MD, FACC, FSCAI Director, Interventional Cardiology Fellowship Program, Banner Good Samaritan Medical Center, Phoenix, Arizona

Stéphane Rinfret, MD, SM, FRCPC, FSCAI Interventional cardiology, Quebec Heart and Lung Institute, Laval University, Quebec, Canada

Rajesh Sachdeva, MD Director, Cardiovascular Medicine, North Fulton Hospital, Roswell, Georgia

Kendrick Shunk, MD, PhD, FACC, FAHA, FSCAI Professor of Clinical Medicine, University of California, San Francisco; Director of Interventional Cardiology, Veterans Affairs Medical Center, San Francisco, California

George Sianos, MD, PhD, FESC Professor, AHEPA University Hospital, Thessaloniki, Greece

Elliot Smith, MD, MRCP London Chest Hospital, Barts Health NHS Trust, London, United Kingdom

James C. Spratt, BSc, MD, FRCP, FESC, FACC Consultant Cardiologist, Forth Valley Royal Hospital, Larbert, United Kingdom

Craig A. Thompson MD, MMSc Director, Interventional Cardiology and Vascular Medicine, Yale University School of Medicine, New Haven, Connecticut

Thomas T. Tsai, MD, MSc Interventional Cardiology, Institute for Health Research, Kaiser Permanente Colorado, Denver, Colorado

Etsuo Tsuchikane, MD, PhD Department of Cardiology, Toyohashi Heart Center, Aichi, Japan

Barry F. Uretsky, MD Director, Interventional Cardiology, University of Arkansas for Medical Sciences and Central Arkansas Veterans Health System, Little Rock, Arkansas

Minh N. Vo University of Manitoba, St. Boniface Hospital Cardiac Science Program, Winnipeg, Canada

Simon J. Walsh, MD, FRCP Consultant Cardiologist, Belfast Health & Social Care Trust; Honorary Lecturer in Cardiology, Queen's University Belfast, Belfast, Ireland

Gerald S. Werner, MD, PhD, FESC, FACC, FSCAI Direktor, Medizinische Klinik I, Klinikum Darmstadt GmbH

R. Michael Wyman, MD Director, Cardiac Catheterization Laboratory and Cardiovascular Interventional Research, Torrance Memorial Medical Center, Torrance, California

Masahisa Yamane, MD, FACC Saitamasekishinkai Hospital and St. Luke's International Hospital, Japan, OLV Cardiovascular Center, Aalst, Belgium

Foreword

The holy grail of interventional cardiology has been to open chronic totally occluded (CTO) coronary arteries. The inability to be predictably successful has been a leading cause of why patients are referred to surgery or left on medical therapy rather than receiving percutaneous revascularization. From the time of Gruentzig and Hartzler, many champions have tried to improve the success rates of opening occluded coronary arteries. In the last 15 years, with the introduction of stiffer guidewires, retrograde techniques, and now antegrade dissection/re-entry techniques, this "holy grail" is now being achieved by a growing number of interventionalists around the globe.

The path to development of all these new technologies and techniques was through collaboration. The initial Japanese experts spent their time teaching others and showing them how to use new wires and retrograde techniques. Further innovation was developed as others saw weaknesses and strengths in early approaches. New technologies and techniques were tried and adapted until a wide array of technical options were available, yet no plan of how and when to use them was offered to those trying to learn. This led to an international group working together to bring an algorithmic approach to CTO percutaneous coronary intervention (PCI) and to show how to embrace new therapies, so that these techniques could be taught.

As you read through the following text you will see many of the "rules" of interventional cardiology being rewritten as a new sub-subspecialty has developed. The language at times will seem foreign, and you will need to learn to be not an interventional cardiologist but a CTO interventionalist. Instead of reviewing angiograms and deciding only whether a patient should get revascularization (either surgically or percutaneously) or medical therapy, you will instead look at the ischemic burden and the patient's symptoms and use the angiogram to determine how to best achieve revascularization. Your skills will grow as you learn to use the subintimal space as your friend, and you will become more efficient, safer, and successful. You will see how retrograde techniques improve your skills and open a host of cases that can now be easily and quickly revascularized.

Medicine is increasingly becoming focused on percutaneous techniques such as TAVR, Mitraclip, left atrial appendage closure, and a host of upcoming therapies aimed at achieving surgical outcomes. But as more less-invasive therapies are used, there will be increasing pressure to achieve success in the one area of interventional cardiology that has lagged behind the surgical cohort, i.e., percutaneous revascularization. Enjoy the journey on a new path to improving your patients' outcomes and your technical skills, and join a new community within interventional cardiology. This community wants to see you succeed, develop skills, and work collaboratively, so that we can all continue to improve our techniques and improve our patients' lives.

William Lombardi, MD

1 CTO Interventions: Definition, Prevalence, Indications, Guidelines

1.1 CTO Definition

Coronary chronic total occlusions (CTOs) are defined as 100% occlusions in the coronary arteries with TIMI 0 flow of at least 3 months' duration.[1] The duration may be difficult to determine if there is no prior angiogram demonstrating presence of the CTO. In such cases estimation of the occlusion duration is based upon first onset of angina or dyspnea and/or prior history of myocardial infarction in the target vessel territory.

Importantly, occluded arteries within 30 days of causing a myocardial infarction, such as those included in the Open Artery Trial (OAT)[2] do not fall within the definition of a CTO. Hence, the lack of benefit observed with percutaneous coronary intervention (PCI) in these subacute lesions should not be extrapolated to CTO patients.

1.2 Prevalence of CTOs

Coronary CTOs are common. In the best contemporary estimate of CTO prevalence at least one coronary CTO was present in 18.4% of patients with coronary artery disease among 14,439 patients undergoing coronary angiography at three Canadian centers.[3] The CTO prevalence was higher (54%) among patients with prior coronary artery bypass graft (CABG) surgery and lower among patients undergoing primary PCI for acute ST-segment elevation myocardial infarction (10%) (Figure 1.1). Left ventricular function

Manual of Coronary Chronic Total Occlusion Interventions. DOI: http://dx.doi.org/10.1016/B978-0-12-420129-3.00001-5

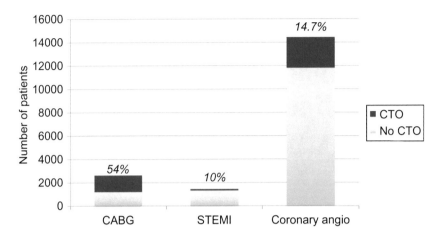

Figure 1.1 Prevalence of coronary CTO in a large multicenter Canadian registry among patients with prior coronary artery bypass graft surgery (CABG), patients with ST-segment elevation acute myocardial infarction (STEMI) and patients undergoing diagnostic coronary angiography.[3] *Source*: Reproduced with permission from Ref. 3.

was normal in >50% of patients with CTO and half of the CTOs were located in the right coronary artery.

Kahn reported a CTO prevalence of 35%, while Werner et al. demonstrated a prevalence of 33% among patients with coronary artery disease (CAD) (defined as ≥50% diameter stenosis in ≥1 vessel) presenting with stable angina.[4,5] Christofferson et al.[6] reported a CTO prevalence of 52% in patients with CAD (defined as ≥70% stenosis in ≥1 vessel) among all non-CABG patients presenting for diagnostic angiography in a registry of 8004 veterans over a 10-year period.

1.3 Indications and Potential Clinical Benefits of CTO PCI

Deciding to perform CTO PCI should depend on the patient's clinical presentation and risk benefit ratio and not the patient's anatomy, as experienced operators using contemporary CTO PCI techniques can be expected to be successful in the great majority of patients

(80−90%), even among the most complex CTO lesions. Successful CTO PCI can provide numerous benefits:

1. **Improve symptoms, such as angina and dyspnea.**
2. **Decrease the need for CABG surgery.**
3. **Decrease the need for anti-anginal medications.**
4. **Reduce mortality (compared to patients with failed CTO PCI).**
5. **Improve left ventricular function.**
6. **Decrease the risk for arrhythmias.**
7. **Improve tolerance of acute coronary syndromes that may occur in the future.**

1. *Improved quality of life*: Successful CTO PCI can decrease or eliminate angina[7,8] and non-anginal[9] symptoms and improve exercise capacity.[10] Joyal et al.[8] performed a meta-analysis comparing patients in whom CTO PCI failed to those in whom CTO PCI was successful. Patients with a successful procedure had significant reductions in recurrent angina during 6 years of follow-up (odds ratio, 0.45; 95% confidence interval, 0.30−0.67).[8] Successful CTO PCI also significantly improved the patients' functional status and quality of life.[7] Apart from angina, many patients with coronary CTOs may present with dyspnea or fatigue. Patients with these manifestations of coronary ischemia are frequently miscategorized as asymptomatic, as patients get accustomed to these symptoms and may not report them, or may minimize their severity. Many patients may also substantially curtail their physical activities and misattribute these adverse lifestyle changes to normal aging or other factors.

2. *Decreased need for CABG (and offer revascularization options to patients who are poor candidates for CABG)*: In patients with stable coronary disease, CABG can reduce mortality and the risk of myocardial infarction in patients with very complex anatomy, whereas outcomes are similar with PCI and CABG in patients with less complex disease (Syntax score ≤22).[11] Thus, CABG is the preferred revascularization modality in patients with complex coronary artery disease. However, many patients decline CABG for nonmedical reasons or because of concerns regarding complications and recovery. Other patients have increased risk for complications if they undergo CABG (e.g., patients with multiple comorbidities or patients who require redo CABG). In such cases, CTO PCI provides additional treatment options. Examples where CTO PCI is preferable to CABG include patients with single vessel right coronary artery CTO and intractable, medically

refractory angina and patients with prior CABG, especially if they have a patent left internal mammary artery graft to the left anterior descending artery.

3. *Decreased need for anti-anginal medications*: Patients who undergo successful CTO PCI usually require fewer or no anti-anginal medications, obviating the medication-related cost and side effects. Eliminating nitrate intake can also allow patients to take phosphodiesterase inhibitors (e.g., sildenafil, vardenafil, tadalafil) for erectile dysfunction.

4. *Reduced mortality*: Whether CTO PCI improves survival is unproven, yet most (but not all[12]) observational studies have shown better survival among patients with successful versus failed CTO PCI[8,13,14] (Figure 1.2), even though bare metal stents or balloon angioplasty were used in many of those studies.

   In a single-center, retrospective study, mortality benefit was only observed when the CTO target vessel was the left anterior descending artery but not the right coronary artery or the circumflex (Figure 1.3).[16]

   Complete revascularization has been associated with lower risk for death, myocardial infarction, and repeat revascularization compared to incomplete revascularization.[17] The presence of a CTO is strongly associated with incomplete revascularization,[18] which in turn is associated with worse clinical outcomes.[19,20] In a study of 301 patients who underwent myocardial perfusion imaging before and after CTO PCI, a baseline ischemic burden of $>12.5\%$ was optimal in identifying patients most likely to have a significant decrease in ischemic burden post−CTO PCI. Hence, the highest benefit of CTO PCI is more likely to be achieved in patients with significant baseline myocardial ischemia.[21]

   Well-developed collateral circulation to the CTO target vessel does not necessarily suggest that ischemia is absent. When fractional flow reserve (FFR) was performed in 92 patients immediately after CTO crossing with a microcatheter but before balloon angioplasty and stenting, FFR was <0.80 in all patients.[22] Similar findings were observed in a study of 50 CTO patients, in which all patients were ischemic regardless of the presence and extent of collateral circulation (Figure 1.4).[23]

5. *Improved left ventricular systolic function*: Successful CTO revascularization can improve left ventricular systolic function,[24−32] provided that the CTO-supplied myocardium is viable[29,30] and the vessel remains patent during follow-up.[27,28]

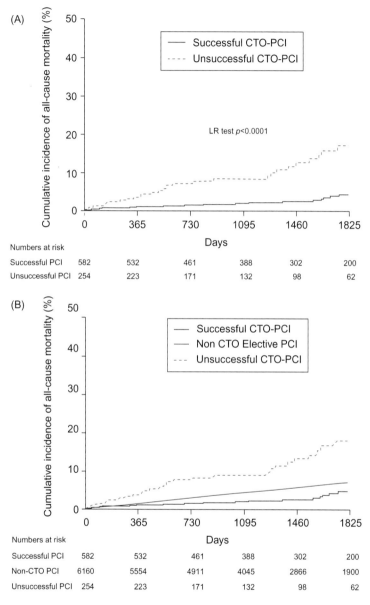

Figure 1.2 Impact of successful CTO revascularization on long-term survival.

Kaplan−Meier curves showing cumulative probability of all-cause mortality after PCI (A) according to procedural success and (B) comparing CTO and non−CTO PCI.

Source: Reproduced with permission from Ref. 15.

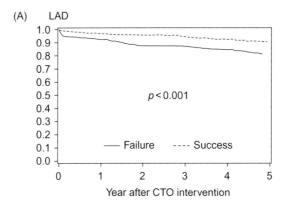

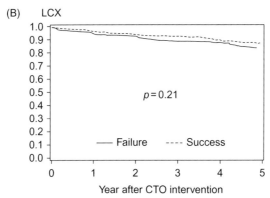

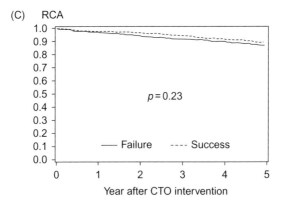

Figure 1.3 Survival between successful and failed CTO PCI among different CTO target vessels. Improved survival was observed if the target vessel was the left anterior descending artery (A), but not if it was the circumflex (B) or the right coronary artery (C).
Source: Reproduced with permission from Ref. 16.

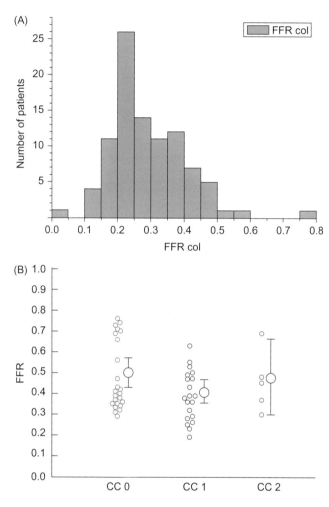

Figure 1.4 Fractional flow reserve after CTO crossing. (A) Fractional flow reserve among 92 CTO patients demonstrating ischemia in all patients. (B) Fractional flow reserve among 50 CTO patients demonstrating ischemia in all patients, even in the presence of well-developed collaterals.
Sources: (A) Courtesy of Dr. Gerald Werner. (B): Reproduced with permission from Ref. 23.

> **Note**
>
> *Viability can be assessed using several techniques; however, if the affected myocardial segment is hypokinetic but not akinetic and if there are no Q-waves in the corresponding region of the electrocardiogram,[33] then viability is highly likely.*

6. Decreased risk for arrhythmias: Ischemia may predispose to ventricular arrhythmias. Among 162 patients with ischemic cardiomyopathy who received an implantable cardioverter defibrillator in the VACTO study, 44% had at least one CTO.[34] During a median follow-up of 26 months, the presence of CTO was associated with higher rates of ventricular arrhythmia and death ($p < 0.01$).[34] However, there is currently no prospective study demonstrating that CTO PCI decreases the risk for subsequent arrhythmias.

7. Improved tolerance of a future acute coronary syndrome: Patients with CTO who develop an acute coronary syndrome (ACS) have much worse outcomes than those who do not have a CTO including patients with multivessel coronary artery disease[35–38] (Figure 1.5).

Although there are no prospective studies showing that "prophylactic" CTO PCI can improve the outcomes of future ACS, a retrospective study showed improved outcomes with successful versus failed CTO PCI after primary PCI for acute ST-segment elevation myocardial infarction (MI).[39]

In addition to the above-mentioned patient benefits, CTO PCI also enhances the operator's overall PCI skills and can improve the success, safety, and efficiency of non−CTO PCI cases. For example, a knuckle wire and a Stingray balloon (described in Section 2.5.2) were used to reenter into the distal true lumen after dissection and guidewire position loss occurred during non−CTO PCI (Figure 1.6).[40] In another case, the Stingray balloon and wire were used to cross the culprit lesion in a patient with ST-segment elevation acute myocardial infarction.[41] Finally, similar devices to those used in coronary CTOs are used to treat peripheral CTOs (such as the Viance catheter and Enteer balloon and guidewires, Covidien) and coronary CTO PCI experience could enhance the outcomes of peripheral arterial interventions.

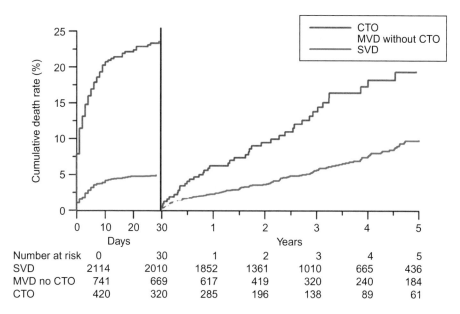

Figure 1.5 Impact of the presence of CTO on outcomes of patients presenting with ST-segment elevation acute myocardial infarction. *Source*: Reproduced with permission from Ref. 36.

1.4 Guidelines for CTO PCI

In the 2011 American College of Cardiology/American Heart Association PCI guidelines, CTO PCI carries a class IIA (level of evidence B) recommendation (Figure 1.7).[42] The guidelines emphasize the importance of selecting patients with appropriate clinical indications for CTO PCI and the importance of operator expertise.

1.5 Appropriateness Use Criteria in CTO PCI

Traditionally CTO PCI has been associated with lower success and higher procedural complication rates; hence, the appropriateness use criteria currently provide lower level recommendation for performing CTO compared to non−CTO PCI (Figure 1.8).[43]

However, with increasing procedural success and decreasing major complication rates with the use of contemporary CTO PCI techniques (Figure 1.9),[44] the appropriateness use criteria for CTO PCI will likely be revised to reflect those advances.

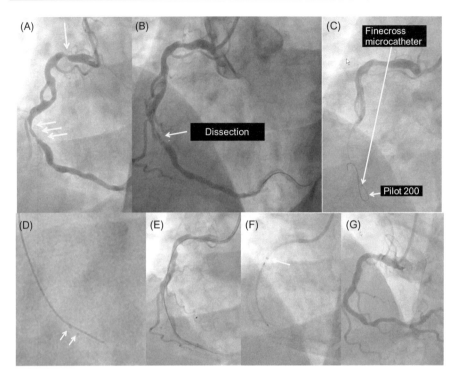

Figure 1.6 Example of CTO techniques application for the treatment of non−CTO lesions. Coronary angiography demonstrating a tortuous right coronary artery with a proximal (arrow, A) and mid (multiple arrows, A) lesions. Mid right coronary artery dissection after balloon predilation (arrow, B). Guidewire position and antegrade flow were lost after an unsuccessful attempt for stent delivery. After failure to advance a guidewire through the dissected segment, a knuckle was formed with a Pilot 200 guidewire (Abbott Vascular) (arrow, C) and advanced around the dissected segment. Using a Stingray balloon (Bridgepoint Medical) (arrows, D) and guidewire distal true lumen re-entry was achieved (D). Using a Guideliner catheter (Vascular Solutions, Minneapolis, MN) (arrow, F) two stents were successfully delivered with an excellent final angiographic result (G). *Source*: Reproduced with permission from Ref. 40.

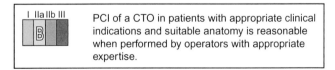

| I IIa IIb III | PCI of a CTO in patients with appropriate clinical indications and suitable anatomy is reasonable when performed by operators with appropriate expertise. |

Figure 1.7 Current American College of Cardiology/American Heart Association guideline recommendation for CTO PCI.

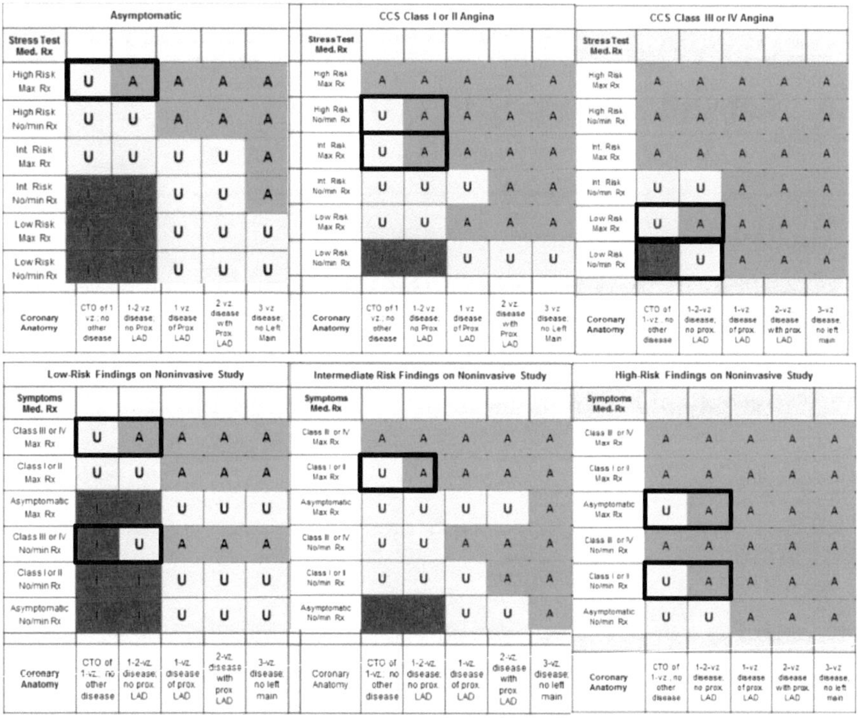

Figure 1.8 Appropriateness use criteria for PCI highlighting categories (10 of 36) in which CTO PCI carries lower recommendation than non−CTO PCI. *Source*: Modified with permission from Ref. 43.

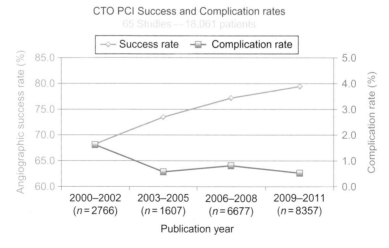

Figure 1.9 Meta-analysis of procedural success and complication rates of CTO PCI, demonstrating increasing success and decreasing complication rates over time. *Source*: Modified with permission from Ref. 44.

1.6   Contraindications to CTO PCI

Absolute contraindications:

1. Inability to receive dual antiplatelet therapy (e.g., due to bleeding diathesis). Patients with contraindications to dual antiplatelet therapy are best treated with CABG surgery.
2. Prior radiation skin injury.

Relative contraindications:

1. Inability to receive prolonged dual antiplatelet therapy required after drug-eluting stent implantation, given the high restenosis rates with bare metal stents in CTOs (as described in Chapter 11).
2. Chronic kidney disease, as high contrast volume may be needed during the procedure (however, contrast use can be minimized using intravascular ultrasonography for PCI guidance or using the retrograde approach).
3. Prior radiation exposure, or multiple and prolonged prior cardiac procedures requiring fluoroscopy, given the increased risk for radiation skin injury with repeat X-ray exposure.
4. Heparin-induced thrombocytopenia (although bivalirudin could potentially be used in such cases).

1.7   Summary and Conclusions

In summary, CTO PCI can provide significant patient benefits when clinically indicated. In symptomatic patients, the myocardium supplied by a CTO is always an ischemic zone, even with well-developed collateral circulation. Continued ischemia is associated with worse clinical outcomes, and successful CTO PCI is important for achieving complete coronary revascularization. How to successfully and safely perform CTO PCI will be discussed in detail in the following chapters.

References

1. Stone GW, Kandzari DE, Mehran R, et al. Percutaneous recanalization of chronically occluded coronary arteries: a consensus document: part I. *Circulation* 2005;**112**: 2364−72.
2. Hochman JS, Lamas GA, Buller CE, et al. Coronary intervention for persistent occlusion after myocardial infarction. *N Engl J Med* 2006;**355**:2395−407.
3. Fefer P, Knudtson ML, Cheema AN, et al. Current perspectives on coronary chronic total occlusions: the canadian multicenter chronic total occlusions registry. *J Am Coll Cardiol* 2012;**59**:991−7.
4. Kahn JK. Angiographic suitability for catheter revascularization of total coronary occlusions in patients from a community hospital setting. *Am Heart J* 1993;**126**:561−4.
5. Werner GS, Gitt AK, Zeymer U, et al. Chronic total coronary occlusions in patients with stable angina pectoris: impact on therapy and outcome in present day clinical practice. *Clin Res Cardiol* 2009;**98**:435−41.
6. Christofferson RD, Lehmann KG, Martin GV, Every N, Caldwell JH, Kapadia SR. Effect of chronic total coronary occlusion on treatment strategy. *Am J Cardiol* 2005;**95**:1088−91.
7. Grantham JA, Jones PG, Cannon L, Spertus JA. Quantifying the early health status benefits of successful chronic total occlusion recanalization: results from the Flowcardia's approach to chronic total occlusion recanalization (FACTOR) Trial. *Circ Cardiovasc Qual Outcomes* 2010;**3**:284−90.
8. Joyal D, Afilalo J, Rinfret S. Effectiveness of recanalization of chronic total occlusions: a systematic review and meta-analysis. *Am Heart J* 2010;**160**:179−87.
9. Safley DM, Grantham J, Jones PG, Spertus J. Health status benefits of angioplasty for chronic total occlusions—an analysis from the OPS/PRISM studies. *J Am Coll Cardiol* 2012;**59** E101.
10. Olivari Z, Rubartelli P, Piscione F, et al. Immediate results and one-year clinical outcome after percutaneous coronary interventions in chronic total occlusions: data from a multicenter, prospective, observational study (TOAST-GISE). *J Am Coll Cardiol* 2003;**41**:1672−8.
11. Mohr FW, Morice MC, Kappetein AP, et al. Coronary artery bypass graft surgery versus percutaneous coronary intervention in patients with

      three-vessel disease and left main coronary disease: 5-year follow-up of
      the randomised, clinical SYNTAX trial. *Lancet* 2013;**381**:629−38.
12.   Yamamoto E, Natsuaki M, Morimoto T, et al. Long-term outcomes
      after percutaneous coronary intervention for chronic total occlusion
      (from the CREDO-Kyoto registry cohort-2). *Am J Cardiol* 2013;**112**
      (6):767−74.
13.   Khan MF, Wendel CS, Thai HM, Movahed MR. Effects of percutane-
      ous revascularization of chronic total occlusions on clinical outcomes:
      a meta-analysis comparing successful versus failed percutaneous inter-
      vention for chronic total occlusion. *Catheter Cardiovasc Interv*
      2013;**82**:95−107.
14.   Muramatsu T, Hiranom K, Tsukahara R, et al. Long-term outcome of
      percutaneous transluminal coronary intervention for chronic total occlu-
      sion in the BMS era in Japan. *Cardiovasc Interv Ther* 2010;**25**:78−84.
15.   Jones DA, Weerackody R, Rathod K, et al. Successful recanalization of
      chronic total occlusions is associated with improved long-term survival.
      JACC Cardiovasc Interv 2012;**5**:380−8.
16.   Safley DM, House JA, Marso SP, Grantham JA, Rutherford BD.
      Improvement in survival following successful percutaneous coronary
      intervention of coronary chronic total occlusions: variability by target
      vessel. *JACC Cardiovasc Interv* 2008;**1**:295−302.
17.   Garcia S, Sandoval Y, Roukoz H, et al. Outcomes after complete ver-
      sus incomplete revascularization of patients with multivessel coronary
      artery disease: a meta-analysis of 89,883 patients enrolled in random-
      ized clinical trials and observational studies. *J Am Coll Cardiol* 2013.
      [published online before print].
18.   Farooq V, Serruys PW, Garcia-Garcia HM, et al. The negative impact
      of incomplete angiographic revascularization on clinical outcomes and
      its association with total occlusions: the SYNTAX (Synergy between
      percutaneous coronary intervention with taxus and cardiac surgery)
      trial. *J Am Coll Cardiol* 2013;**61**:282−94.
19.   Hannan EL, Wu C, Walford G, et al. Incomplete revascularization in
      the era of drug-eluting stents: impact on adverse outcomes. *JACC
      Cardiovasc Interv* 2009;**2**:17−25.
20.   Genereux P, Palmerini T, Caixeta A, et al. Quantification and impact
      of untreated coronary artery disease after percutaneous coronary inter-
      vention: the residual SYNTAX (Synergy between PCI with taxus and
      cardiac surgery) score. *J Am Coll Cardiol* 2012;**59**:2165−74.
21.   Safley DM, Koshy S, Grantham JA, et al. Changes in myocardial ische-
      mic burden following percutaneous coronary intervention of chronic
      total occlusions. *Catheter Cardiovasc Interv* 2011;**78**:337−43.

22. Werner GS, Surber R, Ferrari M, Fritzenwanger M, Figulla HR. The functional reserve of collaterals supplying long-term chronic total coronary occlusions in patients without prior myocardial infarction. *Eur Heart J* 2006;**27**:2406−12.

23. Sachdeva R, Agrawal M, Flynn SE, Werner GS, Uretsky BF. The myocardium supplied by a chronic total occlusion is a persistently ischemic zone. *Catheter Cardiovasc Interv* 2013. [published online before print].

24. Melchior JP, Doriot PA, Chatelain P, et al. Improvement of left ventricular contraction and relaxation synchronism after recanalization of chronic total coronary occlusion by angioplasty. *J Am Coll Cardiol* 1987;**9**:763−8.

25. Danchin N, Angioi M, Cador R, et al. Effect of late percutaneous angioplastic recanalization of total coronary artery occlusion on left ventricular remodeling, ejection fraction, and regional wall motion. *Am J Cardiol* 1996;**78**:729−35.

26. Van Belle E, Blouard P, McFadden EP, Lablanche JM, Bauters C, Bertrand ME. Effects of stenting of recent or chronic coronary occlusions on late vessel patency and left ventricular function. *Am J Cardiol* 1997;**80**:1150−4.

27. Sirnes PA, Myreng Y, Molstad P, Bonarjee V, Golf S. Improvement in left ventricular ejection fraction and wall motion after successful recanalization of chronic coronary occlusions. *Eur Heart J* 1998;**19**:273−81.

28. Piscione F, Galasso G, De Luca G, et al. Late reopening of an occluded infarct related artery improves left ventricular function and long term clinical outcome. *Heart* 2005;**91**:646−51.

29. Baks T, van Geuns RJ, Duncker DJ, et al. Prediction of left ventricular function after drug-eluting stent implantation for chronic total coronary occlusions. *J Am Coll Cardiol* 2006;**47**:721−5.

30. Kirschbaum SW, Baks T, van den Ent M, et al. Evaluation of left ventricular function three years after percutaneous recanalization of chronic total coronary occlusions. *Am J Cardiol* 2008;**101**:179−85.

31. Cheng AS, Selvanayagam JB, Jerosch-Herold M, et al. Percutaneous treatment of chronic total coronary occlusions improves regional hyperemic myocardial blood flow and contractility: insights from quantitative cardiovascular magnetic resonance imaging. *JACC Cardiovasc Interv* 2008;**1**:44−53.

32. Werner GS, Surber R, Kuethe F, et al. Collaterals and the recovery of left ventricular function after recanalization of a chronic total coronary occlusion. *Am Heart J* 2005;**149**:129−37.

33. Surber R, Schwarz G, Figulla HR, Werner GS. Resting 12-lead electrocardiogram as a reliable predictor of functional recovery after

recanalization of chronic total coronary occlusions. *Clin Cardiol* 2005;**28**:293−7.

34. Nombela-Franco L, Mitroi CD, Fernandez-Lozano I, et al. Ventricular arrhythmias among implantable cardioverter-defibrillator recipients for primary prevention: impact of chronic total coronary occlusion (VACTO Primary Study). *Circ Arrhythm Electrophysiol* 2012;**5**: 147−54.

35. Claessen BE, Dangas GD, Weisz G, et al. Prognostic impact of a chronic total occlusion in a non-infarct-related artery in patients with ST-segment elevation myocardial infarction: 3-year results from the HORIZONS-AMI trial. *Eur Heart J* 2012;**33**:768−75.

36. Claessen BE, van der Schaaf RJ, Verouden NJ, et al. Evaluation of the effect of a concurrent chronic total occlusion on long-term mortality and left ventricular function in patients after primary percutaneous coronary intervention. *JACC Cardiovasc Interv* 2009;**2**:1128−34.

37. Hoebers LP, Vis MM, Claessen BE, et al. The impact of multivessel disease with and without a co-existing chronic total occlusion on short- and long-term mortality in ST-elevation myocardial infarction patients with and without cardiogenic shock. *Eur J Heart Fail* 2013;**15**: 425−32.

38. Lexis CP, van der Horst IC, Rahel BM, et al. Impact of chronic total occlusions on markers of reperfusion, infarct size, and long-term mortality: a substudy from the TAPAS-trial. *Catheter Cardiovasc Interv* 2011;**77**:484−91.

39. Yang ZK, Zhang RY, Hu J, Zhang Q, Ding FH, Shen WF. Impact of successful staged revascularization of a chronic total occlusion in the non-infarct-related artery on long-term outcome in patients with acute ST-segment elevation myocardial infarction. *Int J Cardiol* 2013;**165**: 76−9.

40. Martinez-Rumayor AA, Banerjee S, Brilakis ES. Knuckle wire and stingray balloon for recrossing a coronary dissection after loss of guidewire position. *JACC Cardiovasc Interv* 2012;**5**:e31−2.

41. Azemi T, Fram DB, Hirst JA. Bailout antegrade coronary reentry with the stingray balloon and guidewire in the setting of an acute myocardial infarction and cardiogenic shock. *Catheter Cardiovasc Interv* 2013;**82**: E211−4.

42. Levine GN, Bates ER, Blankenship JC, et al. ACCF/AHA/SCAI Guideline for Percutaneous Coronary Intervention. A report of the American College of Cardiology Foundation/American Heart Association Task Force on Practice Guidelines and the Society for Cardiovascular Angiography and Interventions. *J Am Coll Cardiol* 2011;**58**:e44−e122.

43. Patel MR, Bailey SR, Bonow RO, et al. ACCF/SCAI/AATS/AHA/ASE/ASNC/HFSA/HRS/SCCM/SCCT/SCMR/STS 2012 appropriate use criteria for diagnostic catheterization: a report of the American College of Cardiology Foundation Appropriate Use Criteria Task Force, Society for Cardiovascular Angiography and Interventions, American Association for Thoracic Surgery, American Heart Association, American Society of Echocardiography, American Society of Nuclear Cardiology, Heart Failure Society of America, Heart Rhythm Society, Society of Critical Care Medicine, Society of Cardiovascular Computed Tomography, Society for Cardiovascular Magnetic Resonance, and Society of Thoracic Surgeons. *J Am Coll Cardiol* 2012;**59**:1995–2027.
44. Patel VG, Brayton KM, Tamayo A, et al. Angiographic success and procedural complications in patients undergoing percutaneous coronary chronic total occlusion interventions: a weighted meta-analysis of 18,061 patients from 65 studies. *JACC Cardiovasc Interv* 2013;**6**:128–36.

2 Equipment

One of the most frequently asked questions about chronic total occlusion (CTO) percutaneous coronary intervention (PCI), especially from programs early in the learning curve, is: what equipment do I really need?[1]

Although many operators would like to have everything available, the reality is that equipment cost and space limitations require prioritization. Here are some criteria to use when deciding the "must haves" for CTO PCI:

1. At least one item that fulfills each of the requisite steps in CTO PCI (e.g., septal crossing, wire externalization, and snaring) should be available.
2. The operator should be familiar with the equipment, understand its strengths and limitations, and be willing to actually use it (otherwise it will expire on the shelf, although the latter is desired for complication management equipment, such as covered stents and coils).

Table 2.1 shows a "must have" and "nice to have" checklist for CTO PCI, classifying equipment into 10 categories.[1−4]

2.1 Sheaths

Most high-volume hybrid CTO operators routinely use bilateral 8 Fr femoral 45-cm-long sheaths, which provide better guide catheter support and torquability compared to shorter sheaths. Long sheaths straighten tortuosity in the iliac arteries, facilitating guide catheter manipulation. The 45-cm-length usually allows the tip of the sheath to reach the level of the diaphragm (Figure 2.1). Although there is increased risk of thrombus formation within longer sheaths, this is rarely an issue, especially for retrograde CTO PCI, given the high activated clotting times (ACTs) (>350 s) achieved for this procedure.

Manual of Coronary Chronic Total Occlusion Interventions. DOI: http://dx.doi.org/10.1016/B978-0-12-420129-3.00002-7

Table 2.1 Checklist of Equipment Needed for CTO Interventions

Category No.	Equipment	Must Have	Good to Have
1.	Sheaths		8 Fr 45 cm long sheaths
2.	Guides	• XB/EBU 3.0, 3.5, 3.75, 4.0 • AL1, AL0.75 • JR4 • Y-connector with hemostatic valve (such as Co-pilot or Guardian)	• 90 cm long • Side-hole guides, especially AL1
3.	Microcatheters	• Corsair (150 cm for retrograde—135 cm for antegrade) • Finecross (150 cm for retrograde—135 cm for antegrade) • Small (1.20, 1.25, or 1.5 mm diameter) 20 mm long over-the-wire balloons of 145 cm or longer total length	• Venture • Valet
4.	Guidewires[a]	Fielder XT Confianza Pro 12 Pilot 200 Sion Fielder FC Viper (0.014 tip) or R350 wire (for externalization)	Miracle 3 or 12
5.	Dissection/re-entry equipment	CrossBoss catheter Stingray balloon and wire	
6.	Snares	Ensnare or Atrieve 18−30 mm or 27−45 mm	Amplatz Gooseneck snares

(*Continued*)

Table 2.1 (Continued)

Category No.	Equipment	Must Have	Good to Have
7.	Balloon "uncrossable-undilatable" lesion equipment	Small 20 mm long over-the-wire and rapid-exchange balloons Tornus Guideliner or Guidezilla	Rotablator Laser Angiosculpt
8.	Intravascular imaging	IVUS (any)	IVUS (solid state)
9.	Complication management	Covered stents Coils + delivery microcatheters (such as Renegade or Progreat) Pericardiocentesis tray	
10.	Radiation protection		Radiation scatter shields

[a]For radial operators, 300 cm wires are required because the trapping technique (Section 3.7) cannot be used through a 6 Fr guide catheter for trapping over-the-wire balloons, the CrossBoss catheter, and the Stingray balloon. However, trapping can be performed for the Finecross and the Tornus 2.1 microcatheter through a 6 Fr guide catheter. Alternatively, guidewire extensions (for the Asahi and Abbott guidewires) are needed.
Source: Modified with permission from Ref. 1.

If radial access is obtained, 6 Fr is the largest sheath that can be used in most patients, although 7 Fr can often be used in larger radial arteries. Although radial access and smaller sheath size can reduce the risk for vascular access complications, disadvantages of 6 Fr guides for CTO PCI include:

1. Weaker support than larger guide catheters.
2. Inability to use the trapping technique (Section 3.7) with over-the-wire balloons, the CrossBoss catheter, the Stingray balloon, and the 2.6-Fr Tornus catheter.

A sheathless guide system (Eaucath, Asahi Intecc) is expected to become available in the United States in 2014 and will allow CTO PCI with 8.5 Fr guides through an arterial puncture equivalent to that created by a 6-Fr sheath. An alternative approach that has gained

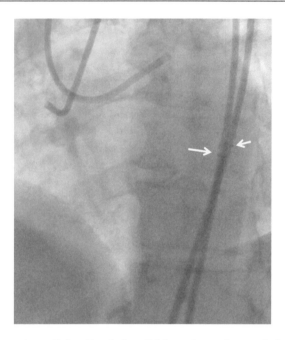

Figure 2.1 Location of the distal tip of 45 cm long femoral sheaths.

popularity among experienced transradial operators is use of regular 8 Fr guides delivered with a sheathless approach. It offers all the advantages of regular 8 Fr catheters and the safety of the transradial approach. The inner and outer diameters of an 8-Fr guide are similar to a 6-Fr sheath. The technique involves introducing a long 110 cm dilator that comes with a long 6 Fr Cook Shuttle sheath into a regular 8 Fr guide. Once the catheter is inserted in the radial artery, the 0.035-in. guidewire is removed, Rotaglide is injected through the dilator, the wire is reintroduced, and the catheter is advanced to the ascending aorta. This technique is similar to the one used for the Asahi EauCath catheters.

2.2   Guide Catheters

2.2.1   Diameter, Length, and Shapes

Dual 8 Fr guides are most commonly used for CTO PCI. Compared to smaller caliber guide catheters, 8 Fr guides provide enhanced support and visualization.

However, even from the femoral approach, the use of 6 Fr guides for the retrograde side can usually provide adequate support for delivering the Corsair catheter and may reduce the risk of donor artery dissection. Therefore, many operators use 6 Fr retrograde catheters from either the femoral or the radial approach. This combination of a 6-Fr radial guide for the retrograde side and an 8-Fr femoral guide for the antegrade side may offer the best of both approaches.

Using 90 cm long guides can facilitate intraprocedural switch to a retrograde approach with wire externalization (100 cm guides can also be used if the Viper or R350 guidewire is available). Shorter (80 cm long) guides may not reach the coronary ostia in some patients and are not commonly used. The "must have" guides are those with supportive shapes, such as the XB, EBU, and AL, for the left coronary artery, and AL and JR4 for the right coronary artery.

2.2.2 Shortening the Guide Catheter

If manufactured short guide catheters are not available, a 100-cm-long guide can be shortened using the following technique (Figure 2.2)[5]:

---

a. The guide catheter is inserted into the body to engage the target coronary artery and the length of the guide that is outside the femoral sheath is marked.

b. The guide is removed from the body and a segment of it is cut, according to the prior measurement (Figure 2.2A).

c. A sheath (1 Fr smaller than the guide catheter, i.e., 6 Fr sheath for a 7 Fr guide catheter) is cut to create a 3- to 4-cm connecting segment for the two guide pieces (Figure 2.2B and C). Both ends of this connecting segment are flared with a dilator (of equal size to the guide) to facilitate insertion (Figure 2.2D).

d. The connecting sheath segment is used to reconnect the proximal and distal guide catheter pieces (Figure 2.2E and F—final result in Figure 2.2G). Placing a Tegaderm (3M) over the connection site may help prevent accidental disconnection.

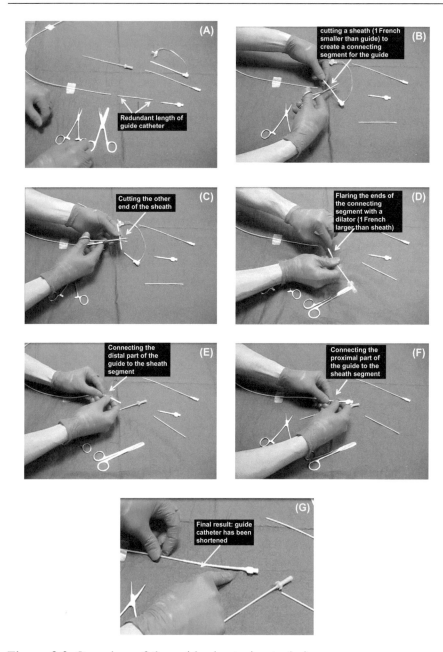

Figure 2.2 Overview of the guide shortening technique.

A limitation of shortened guide catheters is that they have poor torque transmission during vessel engagement and guide manipulations.

2.2.3 Side Holes

For right coronary artery CTOs guide catheters with side holes are commonly used (especially for proximal occlusions) because they prevent pressure dampening, may allow antegrade flow into the vessel, and may decrease the risk for hydraulic dissection during antegrade contrast injection. However, side-hole guides may also provide a false sense of security, as hydraulic dissections can still occur upon injection. Moreover, dampening of the pressure ensures that minimal antegrade flow is provided, when antegrade dissection/re-entry techniques are used.

In contrast, engagement of an unprotected left main coronary artery with side-hole guide catheters should be avoided (with the exception of ostial left main CTOs), because suboptimal guide catheter position may not be recognized and may lead to decrease in antegrade left main flow, resulting in ischemia and hemodynamic collapse. Another disadvantage of side-hole guide catheters is that they lead to higher contrast dose due to escape of part of the contrast into the aorta through the side holes.[3] If no side-hole guides are available, an 18G needle can be used to create side holes in the guide catheter (which may, however, prevent advancement of a guide catheter extension and can weaken the guide and lead to kinking).

2.2.4 Y-Connectors with Hemostatic Valves

CTO PCIs can be lengthy procedures and can be associated with significant blood loss. Using a Y-connector with a hemostatic valve (such as the Co-Pilot, Abbott Vascular, or Guardian, Vascular Solutions) can help minimize blood loss from back bleeding and is easier to use compared with standard rotating hemostatic valves.

2.3   Microcatheters

Antegrade CTO crossing should always be attempted using an over-the-wire system, i.e., a microcatheter or an over-the-wire balloon, because such a system:

---

a. Provides better support and increases the wire tip stiffness, enhancing its penetration capacity (Figure 2.3).
b. Allows reshaping of the guidewire tip.
c. Allows easy guidewire exchanges.
d. Allows accurate assessment of the microcatheter tip location (because the marker is located at the tip, whereas in 1.201.50 mm balloons the marker is located in mid shaft and the tip is not angiographically visible).

Several microcatheters are commercially available (Table 2.2), but four of them are used more commonly in CTO PCI: Corsair (Boston Scientific), Finecross (Terumo), Venture (Vascular Solutions), and Valet (Volcano).

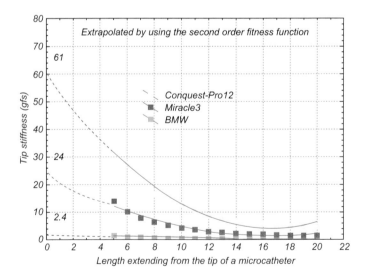

Figure 2.3 Change in guidewire tip stiffness with various guidewire lengths extending past a microcatheter tip.
Source: Reproduced with permission from Ref. 6.

Table 2.2 Overview of Commercially Available Microcatheters

Manufacturer	Catheter	Length	Distal Shaft Outer Diameter
Asahi Intecc	Tornus	135 cm	2.1 and 2.6 Fr
	Corsair	135 cm, 150 cm	2.6 Fr
Boston Scientific	Renegade 18	105 cm, 115 cm, 135 cm	2.5 Fr
	Tracker Excel 14	150 cm	1.9 Fr
	Excelsior 1018	150 cm	2.0 Fr
Cordis	Transit	135 cm	2.5 Fr
	Prowler	150 cm	1.9 Fr
Spectranetics	Quick Cross	135 cm, 150 cm	2.0 Fr
Terumo	Progreat	110 cm, 130 cm	2.4 and 2.7 Fr
	Finecross MG	130 cm, 150 cm	1.8 Fr
Vascular Solutions	Minnie	90 cm, 135 cm, 150 cm	2.2 Fr
	SuperCross	130 cm, 150 cm	2.1 Fr
		With preformed tip angle options of straight, 45°, 90° or 120°	
	Venture	145 cm (rapid exchange) 140 cm (over-the-wire)	2.2 Fr
	Twin Pass 5200	140 cm	1.9 Fr distal tip 3 Fr crossing profile
Volcano	Valet	135 cm 150 cm	1.8 Fr shapeable distal tip

Source: Modified with permission from Ref. 3.

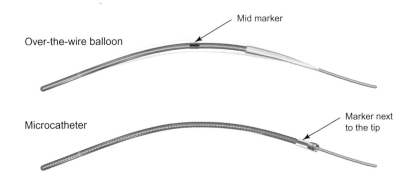

Figure 2.4 Comparison of over-the-wire balloons and microcatheters used for CTO PCI.

2.3.1 Over-the-Wire Balloons

Either a microcatheter or an over-the-wire balloon can be used to support antegrade CTO PCI. In general, microcatheters are preferred because:

a. They allow better understanding of the distal tip position (a marker is placed at the microcatheter tip, whereas in small balloons, the marker is located in the middle of the balloon) (Figure 2.4).
b. They are more flexible and track better than the balloons.
c. They have less tendency to kink than over-the-wire balloons (kinking of the balloon shaft prohibits future wire exchanges and often necessitates balloon catheter and wire removal and replacement with new gear, losing the crossing progress achieved). However, over-the-wire balloons provide better support than most microcatheters.

2.3.2 Corsair

The Corsair microcatheter (Asahi Intecc) was developed as a channel dilator to facilitate retrograde CTO PCI.[7] The Corsair "Shinka" shaft is constructed with eight thin wires wound with two larger wires, which facilitates torque transmission (Figure 2.5). The inner lumen is lined with a polymer that enables contrast injection and facilitates wire advancement. The distal 60 cm of the catheter are coated with a hydrophilic polymer to enhance crossability. The tip is tapered and

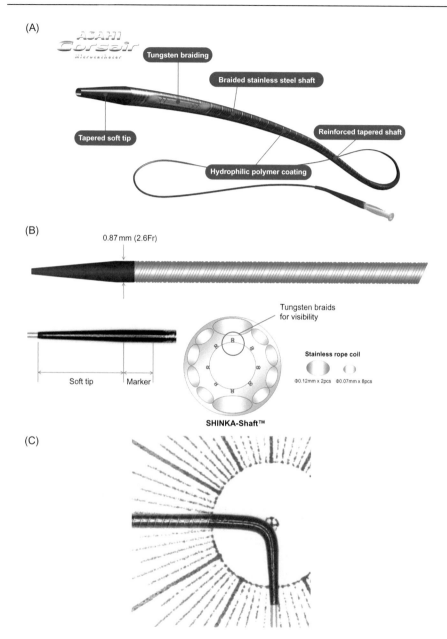

Figure 2.5 Illustration of the Corsair microcatheter. Overview (A) and construction (B) of the Corsair microcatheter. (C) demonstrates the flexibility of the Corsair catheter distal tip.
Source: Reproduced with permission from Asahi Intecc.

soft and is loaded with tungsten powder to enhance visibility. A platinum marker coil is placed 5 mm from the tip.

Corsair: Tips and Tricks

1. Two Corsair lengths are currently available (135 cm long with light blue proximal hub and 150 cm long with dark blue proximal hub).
2. The Corsair can also be used in the antegrade direction for wire support and exchange (usually the 135 cm long Corsair).
3. The Corsair catheter can be advanced by rotating in either direction, although it is braided to have better power when rotated counterclockwise. If resistance is encountered, a counterclockwise rotation associated with forward push is the most powerful maneuver. However, the Corsair should not be over-rotated (>10 consecutive turns without release), as over-rotation could cause catheter deformation and entrapment or fracture proximal to the catheter tip.
4. Rotation of the catheter with both hands and gentle antegrade pressure allows for displacement of friction and tracking along the guidewire. Advancing a Corsair retrogradely across a septal collateral may take several minutes.
5. Contrast can be injected through the Corsair for distal vessel visualization, but the catheter should subsequently be flushed to minimize the risk for guidewire "stickiness." Rarely, the wire may get "stuck" requiring removal of both the Corsair and the guidewire.
6. If difficulty is encountered while attempting to advance the Corsair catheter after prolonged use, the cause may be "Corsair fatigue," and one should consider exchanging for a new Corsair. Also the Corsair tip may become flared and advance poorly, also requiring exchange for a new catheter.
7. If wire externalization is performed, the tip of antegrade equipment (such as balloons and stents) should never come in contact with the tip of the retrograde Corsair catheter over the same guidewire to avoid "interlocking" and equipment entrapment (as described in Chapter 12).

2.3.3 Finecross

The Finecross (Terumo) and Valet (Volcano) microcatheters are the lowest crossing profile microcatheters currently available

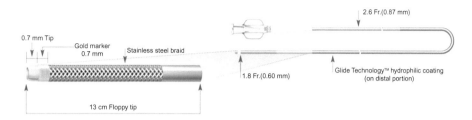

Figure 2.6 Construction of the Finecross catheter.
Source: Reproduced with permission from Terumo Medical.

(1.8 Fr distal tip). The Finecross catheter has a stainless steel braid (to enhance torquability) and a distal marker located 0.7 mm from the tip (Figure 2.6).

Finecross Catheter: Tips and Tricks

1. The Finecross catheter is very flexible and navigates well through tortuosity.
2. Although this catheter is mainly advanced using forward push, many operators are using a combination of push and rotation to facilitate advancement.
3. The Finecross catheter (as well as the Corsair, Venture, and Valet microcatheters) cannot be used for delivering coils. Coil delivery requires a larger microcatheter, such as the Progreat (2.4 Fr, Terumo), Renegade (2.5 Fr, Boston Scientific), and Transit (2.5 Fr, Cordis).

2.3.4 Venture

The Venture catheter (Vascular Solutions, Figure 2.7) has an 8-mm radiopaque torquable distal tip that has a bend radius of 2.5 mm.[8-13] The tip can be deflected up to 90° degrees by clockwise rotation of a thumb wheel on the external handle. With rotation of the entire catheter, steering in all planes is possible. It is compatible with 6 Fr guiding catheters and with 0.014 in. guidewires. Both a rapid exchange and an over-the-wire catheter are available, but the over-the-wire Venture catheter should be used for CTO PCI, as it allows for wire exchanges.

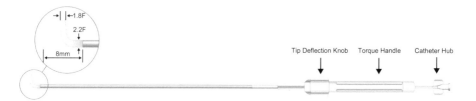

Figure 2.7 Illustration of the over-the-wire Venture catheter.
Source: Reproduced with permission from Vascular Solutions.

Venture: Tips and Tricks

1. The Venture catheter has a deflectable tip, which can be utilized to assist with accessing difficult side branch vessels. As shown in Figure 2.8, the catheter design allows the operator to rotate the tip deflector twist knob in order to transmit increasing tip deflection to the distal tip of the microcatheter.
2. Usually the Venture catheter is delivered to the target vessel in a straight configuration over a workhorse guidewire (Figure 2.9A and B). Once it reaches the target coronary segment the guidewire is withdrawn inside the Venture catheter (Figure 2.9C) and the tip deflector twist knob is clockwise rotated to deflect the catheter tip. The deflected catheter is rotated and withdrawn until it points to the proximal cap (Figure 2.9D), followed by guidewire advancement into the CTO (Figure 2.9E). The Venture catheter can then be removed leaving the guidewire in place in the target vessel (Figure 2.9F).
3. The classic example of Venture catheter use is for treating ostial circumflex CTOs (Figure 2.10).

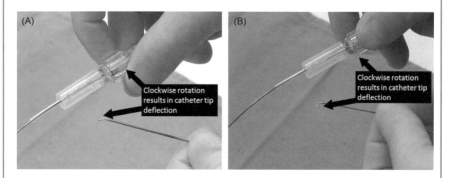

Figure 2.8 Illustration of Venture catheter manipulation.
Source: Courtesy of Dr. William Nicholson.

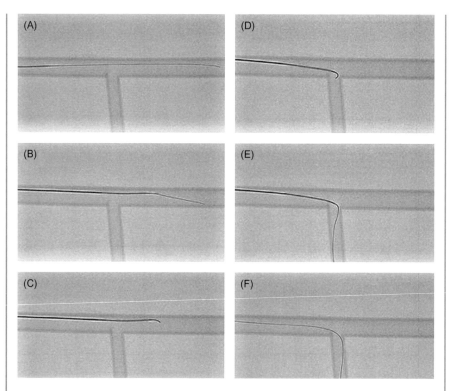

Figure 2.9 Illustration of the use of the Venture catheter.
Source: Courtesy of Dr. William Nicholson.

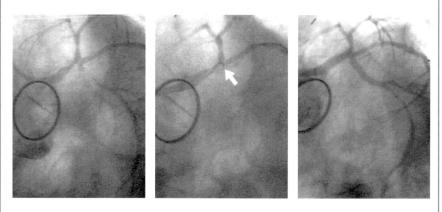

Figure 2.10 Example of Venture catheter use to cross an ostial circumflex CTO.
Source: Reproduced with permission from Ref. 10.

4. The Venture catheter can also prevent the guidewire from prolapsing into a side branch, when CTO penetration is challenging.[14]
5. During retrograde CTO PCI, the Venture catheter can be used to enable wiring of a collateral branch, especially if it arises at an acute angle.
6. Removal of the Venture catheter using a "trapping balloon technique" requires use of a guide catheter that is at least 8 Fr, because the Venture catheter has a larger profile compared to an over-the-wire balloon.[13] For the same reason, an 8-Fr guide catheter is needed to perform a parallel-wire technique, when one of the wires is inserted through the Venture catheter.
7. The Venture catheter is stiff: this can be both an advantage and disadvantage, as it can provide extra support, but can also predispose to target vessel injury. Since the bend radius is 2.5 mm, special care must be exercised when deflecting the tip in <2.5 mm diameter arteries.
8. The Venture catheter bend should be released and the tip straightened before advancing or removing the catheter to prevent vessel damage.

2.3.5 Valet

The Valet microcatheter has a 1.8-Fr distal tip and a 1-mm radiopaque gold marker 0.5 mm from the tip with a hydrophilic coating on the distal 30 cm. It has a shapeable distal tip, excellent torque transmission and provides strong guidewire support (Figure 2.11).

Valet Catheter: Tips and Tricks

1. The catheter tip should be shaped using only fingers by gently stroking the tip between the forefinger and the thumb. The tip should not be shaped with an external object, such as a needle introducer.
2. Contrast can be injected through the Valet for vessel visualization, but the catheter should subsequently be flushed to minimize the risk for guidewire "stickiness."

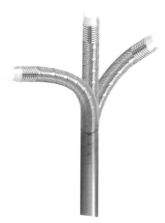

Figure 2.11 Illustration of the Valet microcatheter, demonstrating how the distal tip can be shaped into different configurations.
Source: Reproduced with permission from Volcano.

2.4 Guidewires

This area has the largest number of options, as well as personal preferences (Table 2.3). However, many high-volume operators advocate limiting the options down to a few "must have" wires (in no particular order) (Figure 2.12):

1. Fielder XT (Asahi Intecc), which is a soft, polymer-jacketed, tapered wire for initial antegrade crossing via microchannels.
2. Confianza Pro 12 (Asahi Intecc), a stiff, tapered tip, penetrating wire, for subsequent attempts, if the course of the vessel is well understood.
3. Pilot 200 (Abbott Vascular), a polymer-jacketed and moderately stiff, non-tapered tip wire, when the course of the target lesion and vessel is uncertain.
4. Sion (hydrophilic, highly torquable soft guidewire with excellent shape retention, Asahi Intecc) or Fielder FC (polymer-jacketed soft wire, Asahi Intecc) for wiring collaterals during retrograde crossing.
5. Viper (335 cm long, CSI) or R350 (350 cm long, Vascular Solutions) wire for externalization.

Table 2.3 Description of Coronary Guidewires Commonly Utilized in CTO PCI

Wire Category	Tip Style	Commercial Name	Tip Stiffness	Manufacturer	Properties
Polymer Covered					
	Tapered	Fielder XT[a]	1.2 g	Asahi Intecc	Front-line wire for antegrade crossing. Can also be used for knuckle wire formation and for retrograde crossing.
	Straight (non-tapered), Low tip stiffness	Fielder FC[a]	1.6 g	Asahi Intecc	Used to cross through collateral vessels during the retrograde approach.
		Whisper LS, MS, ES	0.8, 1.0, 1.2 g	Abbott Vascular	
		Pilot 50	1.5 g	Abbott Vascular	
		Choice PT Floppy	2.1 g	Boston Scientific	
	Straight (non-tapered), High tip stiffness	Pilot 150 | 200[a]	2.7 g|4.1 g	Abbott Vascular	Antegrade crossing, especially when the course of the occluded vessel is unclear. Also useful for knuckle wire formation and for re-entry into true lumen during LAST technique.

Description	Wire	Weight	Manufacturer	Notes
	Crosswire NT	7.7 g	Terumo	
	PT Graphix Intermediate	1.7 g	Boston Scientific	
	PT2 Moderate Support	2.9 g	Boston Scientific	
	Shinobi	7.0 g	Cordis	
	Shinobi Plus	6.8 g	Cordis	
Open Coil (no Polymer jacket)				
Straight, low tip stiffness	SION (hydrophilic)[a]	0.8	Asahi Intecc	First choice guidewire for retrograde crossing.
Tapered, low tip stiffness	Cross-it 100XT (0.010 in.)	1.7 g	Abbott Vascular	
	Runthrough NS Tapered (0.008 in.)	1.0 g	Terumo	
Tapered, high tip stiffness, hydrophilic coating	Confianza Pro 9, 12[a] (0.009")	9.3,12.4 g	Asahi Intecc	Antegrade crossing when vessel course is known.
	PROGRESS 140T, 200T (0.0105", 0.009")	12.5, 13.3 g	Abbott Vascular	
	Persuader 9 (0.011")	9.1 g	Medtronic	
	ProVia 9, 12 (0.009")	11.8, 13.5 g	Medtronic	
	MiracleBros 3, 4.5, 6	3.9, 4.4, 8.8 g	Asahi Intecc	Antegrade crossing when vessel course is known.

(Continued)

Table 2.3 (Continued)

Wire Category	Tip Style	Commercial Name	Tip Stiffness	Manufacturer	Properties
	Straight tip, high tip stiffness	MiracleBros 12	13.0 g	Asahi Intecc	
		PROGRESS 40, 80, 120	5.5, 9.7, 13.9 g	Abbott Vascular	
		Persuader 3, 6 (-philic and –phobic)	5.1, 8.0 g	Medtronic	
		Provia 3, 6 (-philic and –phobic)	8.3, 9.1 g	Medtronic	
	Tapered, high tip Stiffness, hydrophobic coating	Confianza 9 (hydrophobic)	8.6 g	Asahi Intecc	Antegrade crossing when vessel course is known.
		Persuader 9 (hydrophobic)	9.1 g	Medtronic	
		ProVia 9, 12 (hydrophobic)	11.8 g, 13.5 g	Medtronic	
Externalization wires		Viper (0.014 tip)[a]		CSI	335 cm in length.
		RG3		Asahi Intecc	330 cm in length.
		RotaWire Floppy and Extra support	3.6 g	Boston Scientific	325 cm in length.
		R350		Vascular Solutions	350 cm in length.

[a]Most commonly utilized guidewires.
Source: Adapted with permission from Ref. 4.

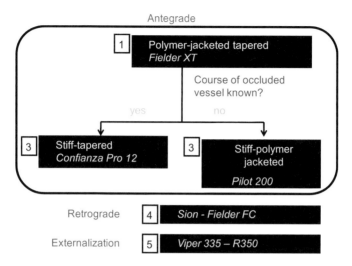

Figure 2.12 Algorithm for guidewire selection.

Except for the retrograde and externalization guidewires many operators currently use only short (180−190 cm) guidewires and remove the microcatheter or over-the-wire balloon using the trapping technique (Section 3.7). However, for operators performing transradial CTO PCI, availability of 300 cm long guidewires and guidewire extensions is important, as the "trapping" technique for exchanging over-the-wire to rapid exchange equipment may not always be feasible through a 6-Fr guide catheter, especially if a guide catheter extension is utilized.

2.4.1   Fielder Guidewires

The Fielder family of guidewires (Figure 2.13, Asahi Intecc) are polymer-jacketed, soft-tip guidewires, with either tapered (Fielder XT, 0.009 in. taper) or non-tapered (Fielder FC) distal tip.

Fielder Guidewires: Tips and Tricks

1. The Fielder XT guidewire is the most commonly used first guidewire for antegrade wire escalation.

2. The Fielder XT is also very useful for forming tight knuckles, both in the antegrade and in the retrograde approaches.

3. The Fielder FC may be useful in antegrade wiring through a visible microchannel, as it may be less likely than the Fielder XT to enter the subintimal space and dissect the microchannel. It is also useful for retrograde crossing via collateral channels, although many operators prefer the Sion as the first choice wire for this purpose.

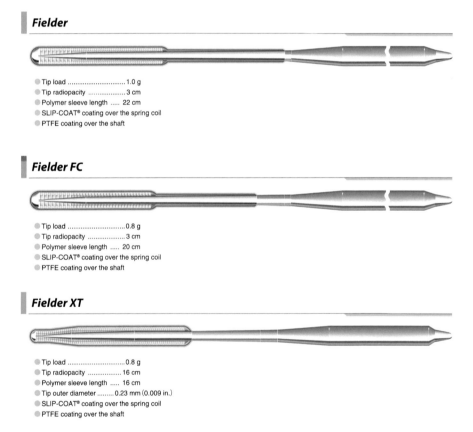

Fielder

- Tip load .... 1.0 g
- Tip radiopacity .... 3 cm
- Polymer sleeve length ..... 22 cm
- SLIP-COAT® coating over the spring coil
- PTFE coating over the shaft

Fielder FC

- Tip load .... 0.8 g
- Tip radiopacity .... 3 cm
- Polymer sleeve length ..... 20 cm
- SLIP-COAT® coating over the spring coil
- PTFE coating over the shaft

Fielder XT

- Tip load .... 0.8 g
- Tip radiopacity .... 16 cm
- Polymer sleeve length ..... 16 cm
- Tip outer diameter .... 0.23 mm (0.009 in.)
- SLIP-COAT® coating over the spring coil
- PTFE coating over the shaft

Figure 2.13 Illustration of the Fielder guidewires.
Source: Reproduced with permission from Asahi Intecc.

2.4.2   MiracleBros and Confianza Family of Wires

The MiracleBros wires (Asahi Intecc) are stiff wires (up to 12 g distal tip stiffness) with high-penetrating power. These wires are nonhydrophilic (hydrophobic) and are favored for delivering gear to CTO segments, caps, or spaces, as they are less likely to slip out of place.

The Confianza guidewires (Asahi Intecc) are stiff but also have a tapered tip (Figure 2.14).

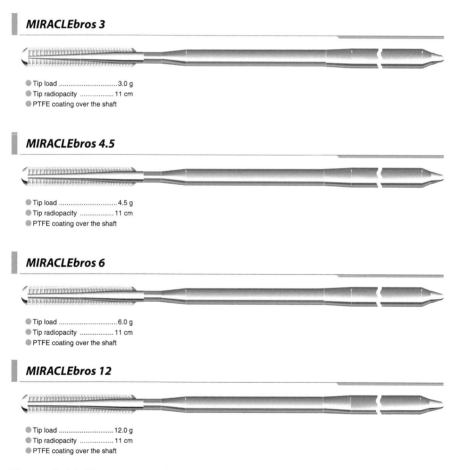

MIRACLEbros 3

- Tip load ....3.0 g
- Tip radiopacity ....11 cm
- PTFE coating over the shaft

MIRACLEbros 4.5

- Tip load ....4.5 g
- Tip radiopacity ....11 cm
- PTFE coating over the shaft

MIRACLEbros 6

- Tip load ....6.0 g
- Tip radiopacity ....11 cm
- PTFE coating over the shaft

MIRACLEbros 12

- Tip load ....12.0 g
- Tip radiopacity ....11 cm
- PTFE coating over the shaft

Figure 2.14 Illustration of the Miracle (A) and Confianza (B) line of wires.
The Confianza wires have tapered tip and the "Pro" wires have hydrophilic coating.
Source: Reproduced with permission from Asahi Intecc.

CONFIANZA

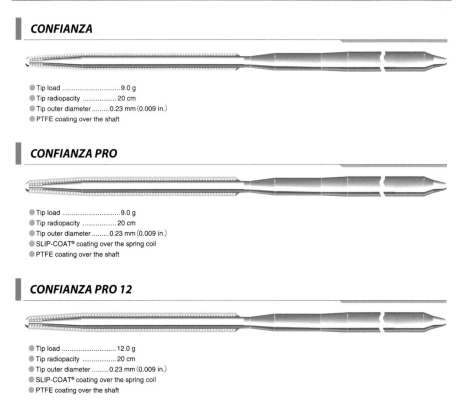

- Tip load ....9.0 g
- Tip radiopacity ....20 cm
- Tip outer diameter ....0.23 mm (0.009 in.)
- PTFE coating over the shaft

CONFIANZA PRO

- Tip load ....9.0 g
- Tip radiopacity ....20 cm
- Tip outer diameter ....0.23 mm (0.009 in.)
- SLIP-COAT® coating over the spring coil
- PTFE coating over the shaft

CONFIANZA PRO 12

- Tip load ....12.0 g
- Tip radiopacity ....20 cm
- Tip outer diameter ....0.23 mm (0.009 in.)
- SLIP-COAT® coating over the spring coil
- PTFE coating over the shaft

Figure 2.14 (*Continued*)

Miracle/Confianza Wires: Tips and Tricks

1. The Confianza Pro 12 guidewire can be very useful in puncturing a calcified proximal CTO cap, given its high-penetrating power.
2. The Confianza Pro 12 guidewire can be very useful when the proximal cap is at the location of a large side branch and initial wires keep deflecting into the side branch. Its stiff tapered tip allows it to be directed away from the side branch to engage and puncture the cap.
3. The Confianza Pro 12 guidewire can also be very useful for re-entering into the true lumen (wire-based re-entry, as described in Chapter 5, Section 4.2).
4. Because of its high-penetrating power, the Confianza Pro 12 wire should not be used in cases where the course of the target CTO vessel is not well understood, as it may easily cause perforation and/or dissection.

> **5.** The MiracleBros wires are very supportive and hydrophobic, with good tactile feedback and are the preferred wires for delivering the Stingray balloon to the re-entry zone, as described in Chapter 5, Section 3).

2.4.3   Pilot Family of Guidewires

Similar to the Fielder guidewires (Asahi Intecc), the Pilot guidewires (Abbott Vascular, Figure 2.15) are polymer-jacketed, but they are stiffer. The Pilot 200 guidewire is a 4.1-g tip guidewire and is the preferred wire for antegrade wire escalation if initial CTO crossing attempts with a soft, tapered polymer-jacketed guidewire fail and/or if the course of the target vessel is not well understood. The Pilot 200 can engage and traverse microchannels, occasionally resulting in true-to-true lumen crossing. It can also be used for knuckle formation both in the antegrade and retrograde direction.

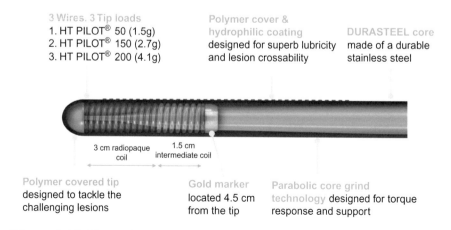

Figure 2.15 Illustration of the Pilot line of wires.
Source: Courtesy of Abbott Vascular. © 2013 Abbott. All rights reserved.

Pilot Wires: Tips and Tricks

1. Although the Pilot 200 is useful for knuckle formation because it is stiffer than Fielder XT, it tends to form a wider knuckle with increased pushability.
2. Because of its transitionless core it has lesser tendency to prolapse into side branches.

2.4.4 Asahi Sion

The Sion guidewire (Asahi Intecc) has a composite core and double-coil technology (Figure 2.16). These features provide excellent torque transmission and resistance to deformation.

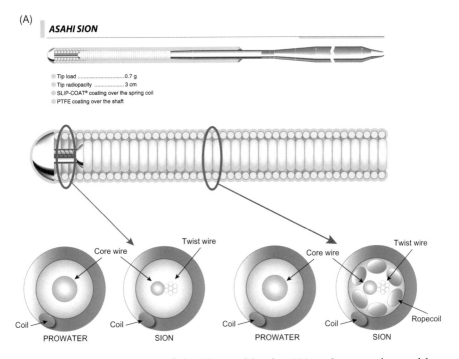

Figure 2.16 Construction of the Sion guidewire (A) and comparison with other Asahi guidewires (B).
Source: Reproduced with permission from Asahi Intecc.

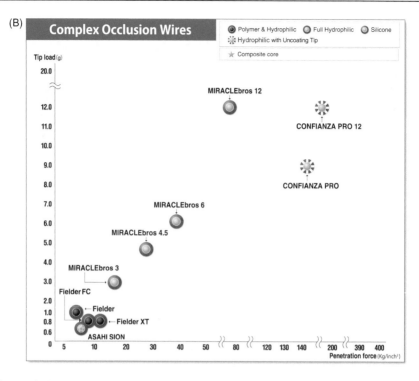

Figure 2.16 (*Continued*)

2.4.5 Externalization Guidewires

Two guidewires are currently used for externalization in the United States during the retrograde approach: the Viper Advance wire (CSI) and the R350 guidewire (Vascular Solutions). The RG3 externalization wire (Asahi Intecc) is not available currently in the United States.

The Viper advance (the 0.014-in. at the tip Viper wire should be used for coronary CTOs, not the 0.017-in. at the tip one), is 335 cm long, and provides excellent support. The R350 (0.013 in.) is 350 cm long and has a 5-cm platinum coil to enhance visualization. The RG3 wire is 330 cm in length, has excellent resistance to kinking, and is the preferred externalization wire outside the United States.

Externalization Wires: Tips and Tricks

1. Externalization is facilitated when the tip of the Corsair (coming from the retrograde guide catheter) is advanced into the antegrade guide catheter.
2. Avoiding wire kinking is very important to facilitate delivery of the externalized guidewire.
3. Administration of a small amount (~0.2 ml) of Rotaglide (Boston Scientific) through the microcatheter can significantly facilitate advancement of the externalization guidewire and is highly recommended prior to introducing the Viper or R350 wires.
4. The wire introducer should be used through the hemostatic valve of the antegrade guide catheter to thread the externalization wire followed by reattachment of the Y-connector to the guide catheter (Chapter 6, Step 8; Figure 6.22).
5. The externalized guidewire can cause significant tissue injury in the collateral circulation if the ends are pulled while the wire is not covered by a microcatheter or over-the-wire balloon.
6. "Managing the loop" (between the guides) and actively maintaining the guide catheter positions is also critical.

2.5 Dissection/Re-Entry Equipment

Even though dissection/re-entry can be accomplished using knuckle wires, the CrossBoss catheter and Stingray balloon and guidewire (Boston Scientific) are preferred, as they improve success rates and procedural efficiency in cases that could not be crossed using standard crossing techniques.

2.5.1 CrossBoss Catheter

The CrossBoss catheter (Figures 2.17 and 2.18) is a stiff, metallic, over-the-wire catheter with a 1-mm blunt, rounded, hydrophilic-coated distal tip that can advance through the occlusion when the catheter is rotated rapidly using a proximal torque device ("fast spin"

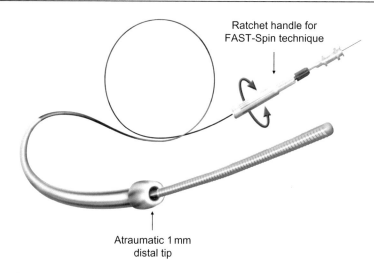

Figure 2.17 Illustration of the CrossBoss catheter.
Source: © 2013 Boston Scientific Corporation or its affiliates. All rights reserved. Used with permission of Boston Scientific Corporation.

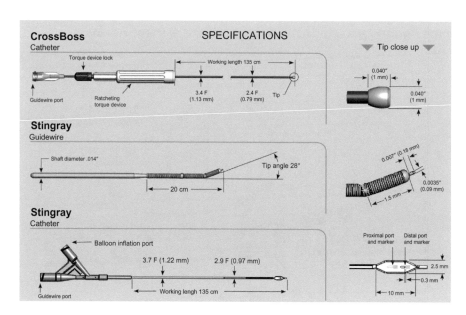

Figure 2.18 Specifications of the CrossBoss catheter and the Stingray balloon and guidewire.
Source: © 2013 Boston Scientific Corporation or its affiliates. All rights reserved. Used with permission of Boston Scientific Corporation.

technique) (Chapter 5). If the catheter enters the subintimal space, it creates a limited dissection plane making re-entry into the distal true lumen easier. The risk of perforation is low, provided that the CrossBoss catheter is not advanced into side branches. If the CTO is crossed subintimally, the Stingray balloon and guidewire can be used to assist with re-entry into the distal true lumen, as described below.[15-17]

2.5.2 Stingray Balloon and Guidewire

The Stingray balloon is 2.5 mm wide when inflated and 10 mm in length and has a flat shape with two-side exit ports. Upon low-pressure (2−4 atm) inflation, it orients one exit port automatically toward the true lumen (Figures 2.18 and 2.19).[18] The Stingray guidewire is a stiff guidewire with a 20-cm distal radiopaque segment and a 0.009-in. tapered tip with a 0.0035-in. distal prong. The Stingray guidewire can be directed toward one of the two side ports of the Stingray balloon under fluoroscopic guidance to re-enter the distal true lumen.[15-17]

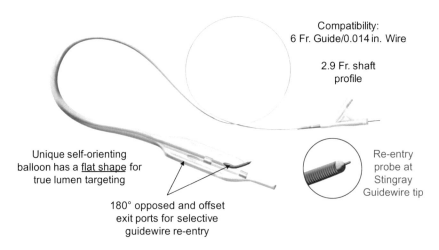

Figure 2.19 Illustration of the Stingray balloon and guidewire.
Source: © 2013 Boston Scientific Corporation or its affiliates. All rights reserved. Used with permission of Boston Scientific Corporation.

CrossBoss and Stingray: Tips and Tricks

1. It is best to avoid advancing stiff guidewires through the CrossBoss catheter, since the CrossBoss greatly enhances the guidewire penetrating power and increases the risk for perforation.
2. The CrossBoss catheter may cross from true-to-true lumen in approximately one-third of the cases.[19]
3. The CrossBoss may be particularly effective for crossing in-stent restenotic CTOs, as the stent struts may act as barrier preventing advancement of the CrossBoss catheter behind the restenosed stent.[20]
4. Inserting the Stingray guidewire into the hub of a balloon or microcatheter should be done using an introducer to prevent deformation of the distal guidewire tip.
5. Extending a knuckled wire dissection plane for the final few centimeters with the CrossBoss will help manage the subintimal space. This minimizes subintimal hematoma formation and helps maintain close proximity to the true lumen at the target re-entry zone, enhancing the likelihood of successful re-entry.
6. In right coronary artery CTOs re-entry should be attempted in a non-tortuous, non-calcified segment closest to the reconstitution zone and proximal to bifurcations if possible.

2.6 Snares

Snares are often needed for gathering the retrograde guidewire into the antegrade guide catheter. Three-loop (tulip) snares, such as the Ensnare (Merit Medical) and the Atrieve (Angiotech), are more effective in capturing the guidewire compared with the single-loop snares, such as the Amplatz Gooseneck snare (Covidien) (Figure 2.20).

2.6.1 Snaring Technique (Figure 2.21)

The snare is withdrawn and collapsed into the introducer tool (Figure 2.21A−C). The snare is then introduced into the antegrade guide catheter (Figure 2.21D and E) and advanced until it exits from the distal guide tip (Figure 2.21F).

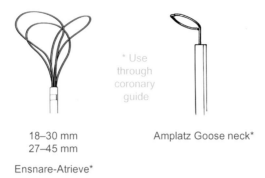

18–30 mm   Amplatz Goose neck*
27–45 mm

Ensnare-Atrieve*

Figure 2.20 Illustration of the three-loop and single-loop snares that are currently commercially available.

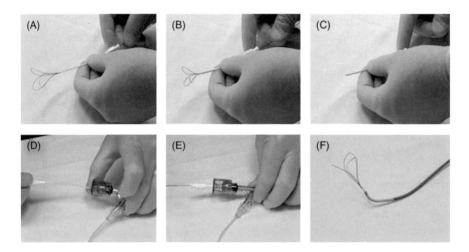

Figure 2.21 Illustration of snare preparation.
Source: Courtesy of Dr. William Nicholson.

The retrograde guidewire is advanced through the snare (Figure 2.22A). The snare is withdrawn into the guide catheter along with the retrograde guidewire (Figure 2.22B–D). The guidewire is pushed through the retrograde guide until it exits from the antegrade guide hub, allowing the antegrade guide to be reseated into the antegrade coronary artery (Figure 2.22E and F).

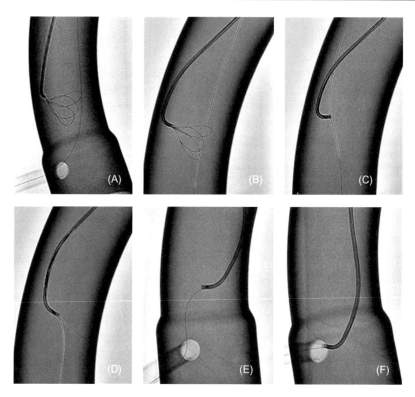

Figure 2.22 Illustration of retrograde guidewire snaring.
Source: Courtesy of Dr. William Nicholson.

Snaring: Tips and Tricks

1. Large snares (27−45 mm or 18−30 mm) are preferred to maximize the likelihood of capturing the retrograde guidewire.
2. Each snare comes with a delivery sheath, which is discarded as the antegrade guide catheter is used for snaring the retrograde guidewire.
3. It is important to not discard the snare-collapsing tool, as it is necessary for re-introducing the snare into the guide catheter, if needed.
4. Ideally, the retrograde microcatheter should be advanced into the aorta before attempting to snare the retrograde guidewire to minimize the risk of the guidewire being retracted back into the CTO.
5. The safest approach to snare the wire that needs externalization (Viper and R350 in the United States and RG3 elsewhere) is on the

radiopaque portion of the wire followed by careful sweeping into the antegrade guide.

6. Alternatively, if a short retrograde guide has been used, some operators prefer to snare 300 cm long Pilot 200 guidewires.

7. Short 180 cm wires should never be snared. If done inadvertently, the wire should be pulled out from the antegrade guide, without attempting to retrieve it from the donor artery direction.

2.7 "Uncrossable-Undilatable" Lesion Equipment

The second most common reason for CTO PCI failure is failure to dilate the lesion after wire crossing. This can be facilitated either by increasing guide catheter support (e.g., using a guide catheter extension and various anchor balloon techniques) or by modifying the lesion by using the Tornus catheter (Asahi Intecc) or various other modalities, such as rotational atherectomy or laser, as described in detail in Chapter 8.

2.7.1 Tornus Catheter

The Tornus catheter (Figure 2.23) consists of eight stainless steel wires stranded in a coil.[21] It comes in two sizes, 2.1 and 2.6 Fr, with the latter providing more guidewire support. It has a platinum marker located 1 mm from the tip. Unlike the Corsair catheter, the Tornus does not have an inner polymer, and as a result, injection of contrast cannot be done through it, but it provides stronger support. The Tornus is advanced by counter-clockwise rotation and withdrawn by clockwise rotation. To avoid catheter kinking and unraveling of the stranded steel wires no more than 20 rotations should be done in any direction.

Tornus Catheter: Tips and Tricks

1. Apart from penetrating "balloon uncrossable" lesions, the Tornus catheter can be used for antegrade wiring, as it provides strong backup support.

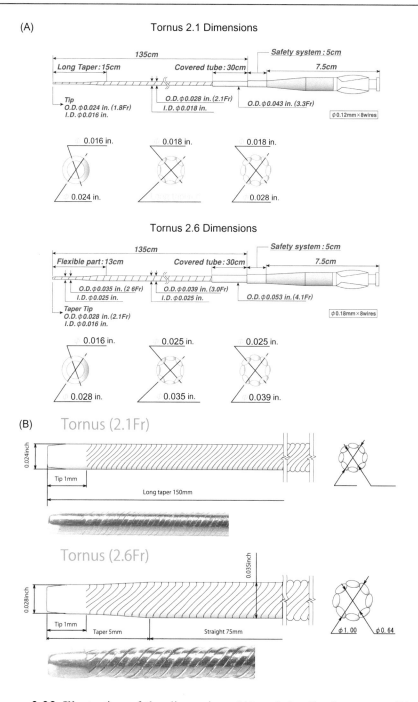

Figure 2.23 Illustration of the dimensions (A) and the distal segment (B) of the Tornus 2.1 and 2.6 catheters.
Source: Reproduced with permission from Asahi Intecc.

2.7.2 Guide Catheter Extensions

Two guide catheter extensions are currently available in the United States: the Guideliner V2 catheter (Vascular Solutions) and the Guidezilla (Boston Scientific).

The Guideliner V2 catheter (Figure 2.24) is a rapid exchange, "mother and child" guide catheter extension that was approved by the

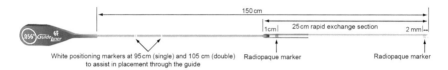

Figure 2.24 Illustration of the Guideliner V2 catheter.
Source: Reproduced with permission from Vascular Solutions.

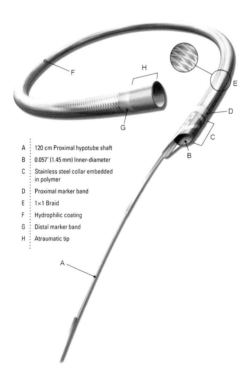

Figure 2.25 Illustration of the Guidezilla catheter.
Source: © 2013 Boston Scientific Corporation or its affiliates. All rights reserved. Used with permission of Boston Scientific Corporation.

FDA in November 2009 and is manufactured in four sizes (5.5, 6, 7, and 8 Fr) that fit through a small 6, 6, 7, and 8 Fr guide catheter, respectively, resulting in an inner diameter that is approximately 1 Fr smaller than that of the guide catheter. It is 145-cm-long and has a 25-cm single lumen cylinder that enters the coronary vessel. It has a radiopaque marker 2.66 mm from the catheter tip.

The Guidezilla catheter (Figure 2.25) is also a rapid exchange, "mother and child" guide catheter extension that was approved by the FDA in March 2013 and is manufactured in one size (6 Fr) that fits though a 6-Fr guide catheter. It is similar to the Guideliner but has slightly larger internal diameter (1.45 mm versus 1.42 mm, respectively).

Guide Catheter Extensions: Tips and Tricks

1. Deformation of stents or other equipment can occur while advancing them through the guide catheter extension collar (Figure 2.26).[22] If this happens, it may be necessary to advance the stent into the guide catheter extension *outside* of the body and advance both as a single unit into the guide catheter.
2. Deformation of stents or other equipment can also occur when withdrawing the equipment back into the distal tip of the catheter after a failed attempt to advance to the target lesion, as shown in Figure 2.27.
3. Deep advancement of the guide catheter extension can cause dissection.[23]
4. During retrograde interventions, a guide catheter extension can be advanced through the antegrade guide catheter to facilitate the reverse Controlled Antegrade and Retrograde Tracking and

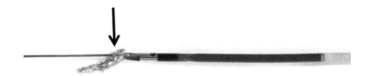

Figure 2.26 Stent deformation while attempting to deliver it through a Guideliner catheter.
Source: Reproduced with permission from Ref. 22.

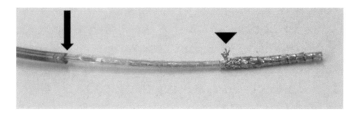

Figure 2.27 Stent deformation while attempting to retrieve an undeployed stent into the distal tip of a Guidezilla catheter. The tip of the Guidezilla prolapsed on itself (arrow) during attempted stent retrieval, resulting in catching the proximal edge of the stent and causing deformation (arrowhead).
Source: Courtesy of Dr. William Nicholson.

Dissection (CART) technique (as described in Chapter 6). The guide extension can also be used from the retrograde side to increase support for Corsair delivery.

5. Every effort should be undertaken to minimize pressure dampening, but if dampening occurs, it is important to verify that adequate antegrade flow is preserved and that no vessel injury has occurred before proceeding with the intervention.[23]

6. Although distal-to-proximal stenting is preferred, "proximal-to-distal" stenting is a viable option by inserting the guide catheter extension through the proximal stent.[24]

7. Advancement of the guide catheter extension into the coronary artery over a balloon catheter or microcatheter is preferred to advancement over a 0.014-in. coronary wire to minimize the risk of catching a plaque edge and causing a dissection.

8. Although co-axial alignment of the guide catheter is ideal, the guide catheter extension may be particularly effective in facilitating vessel engagement and equipment delivery when co-axial alignment is not possible. Distal anchoring may be needed to deliver the guide catheter extension in such cases.[23]

9. The proximal collar of the guide catheter extension should not be advanced outside the guide catheter.

10. Because the guide catheter extensions decrease the original guide size by 1 Fr, special attention to pressure dampening and to the activated clotting time is needed to decrease the risk of thrombus formation.

2.7.3 Angiosculpt

The AngioSculpt® scoring balloon catheter (AngioScore, Inc.) (Figure 2.28) is composed of a semi-compliant balloon encircled by three nitinol spiral struts to score the target lesion on balloon inflation. Compared with the cutting balloon, the Angiosculpt balloon has lower profile and produces more scoring marks per millimeter of plaque.

2.8 Intravascular Ultrasound

Intravascular ultrasound (IVUS) can help:

---

a. Identify the lesion proximal cap in cases with proximal cap ambiguity.

b. Confirm that the antegrade guidewire has engaged the CTO lesion (Figure 2.29).

c. Confirm that the retrograde guidewire has entered the proximal true lumen before externalization.

d. Determine the appropriate balloon size for the CART and reverse CART techniques.

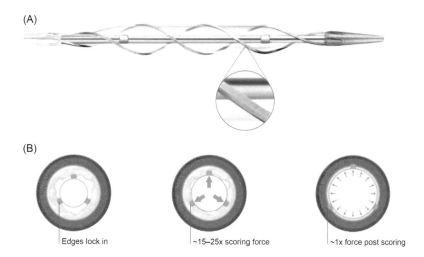

Figure 2.28 Illustration of the Angiosculpt balloon (A) and its mechanism of action (B).
Source: Reproduced with permission from Angioscore.

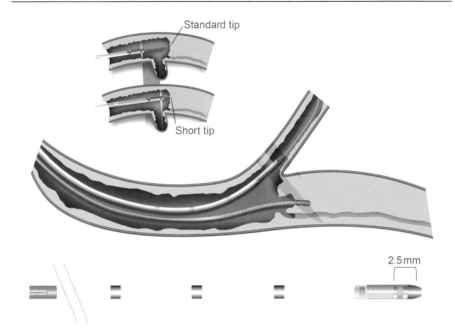

Figure 2.29 Illustration of use of IVUS for guiding the entry of the crossing guidewire into the CTO.
Source: Reproduced with permission from Volcano.

IVUS: Tips and Tricks

1. Solid-state, phased array systems (Eagle Eye, Volcano) are preferred over rotational IVUS systems, such as the Revolution (Volcano), Altantis SR Pro (Boston Scientific), and TVC (InfraRedx) because the imaging transducer is closer to the IVUS catheter tip.
2. A short-tip solid state IVUS catheter was recently introduced in the market (Eagle Eye Short Tip, Volcano, Figure 2.29) and is preferred for imaging during CTO PCI, as it minimizes the extent of distal dissection required for distal imaging and is more deliverable.

2.9 Complication Management Equipment

Although this equipment is rarely needed, it must be available not only for CTO PCI, but also for any other PCI.

2.9.1 Covered Stents

In the United States, there is currently only one coronary covered stent, and it is available with both over-the-wire (Jostent Graftmaster, Abbott Vascular) and rapid exchange (Graftmaster Rx, Abbott Vascular) delivery systems. It is approved through a humanitarian device exemption[25] for use in large vessel perforations (Figure 2.30).

Covered Stents: Tips and Tricks[26]

In general:

a. The Graftmaster consists of two stainless steel stents with a middle layer of ePTFE.

b. It is bulky and difficult to deliver, hence excellent guide catheter support is important.

c. The Graftmaster may be difficult to advance through previously deployed stents, necessitating techniques such as distal anchor and use of guide catheter extensions such as the Guideliner catheter (Vascular Solutions, Minneapolis, MN) (ideally the larger 8 Fr Guideliner).

d. Minimum inflation pressure is 15 atm, but even higher pressures (and use of IVUS) are preferred to ensure adequate stent expansion.

e. After expansion the stent may shorten up to 1.6 mm on each side (for a total of 3.2 mm at nominal pressure—15 atm). Hence, adequate overlap of stents is important to cover long areas of perforation.

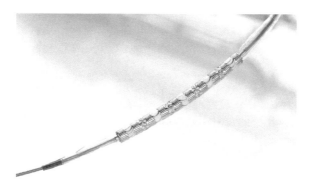

Figure 2.30 Illustration of the Graftmaster Rx covered stent.
Source: Courtesy of Abbott Vascular. © 2013 Abbott. All rights reserved.

f. Use of a *dual catheter ("ping-pong guide") technique* (see Chapter 12, Section 1.1.2.3) is often required to minimize bleeding into the pericardium while preparing for covered stent delivery and deployment.[27]

Rapid exchange system (Graftmaster Rx):
a. Is available in diameters of 2.8–4.8 mm and lengths between 16 and 26 mm.
b. Requires a 6-Fr guide catheter for the 2.8–4.0 mm stents and a 7-Fr guide catheter for the 4.5 and 4.8 mm stents.

Over-the-wire system (Jostent Graftmaster):
a. Is available in diameters of 3.0–5.0 mm and lengths between 9 and 26 mm.
b. Requires a 300-cm-long wire for delivery.
c. Its use will likely decline now that a rapid exchange covered stent (Graftmaster Rx) is available.

2.9.2 Coils

Coils should be available for use in case of distal branch or collateral vessel perforation. Metallic coils are permanent embolic agents that can be deployed through large microcatheters.[28] Coils are usually made of stainless steel or platinum alloys with synthetic wool or Dacron fibers attached along the length of the wire to increase thrombogenicity. Once advanced into the target vessel, the coils assume a preformed shape, sealing the perforation (Figure 2.31).

Coils: Tips and Tricks[26]

a. Given that coils are used very infrequently in cardiac catheterization laboratories, it is important for each operator to be familiar with the principles underlying their use and with 1–2 specific coil types that can be delivered rapidly in case of perforation.
b. Coils cannot be delivered through the usual microcatheters used during CTO PCI (such as the Finecross or Corsair catheter) but require larger microcatheters, such as the Progreat, Renegade, and Transit microcatheters.

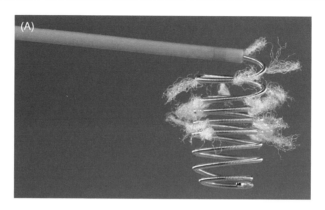

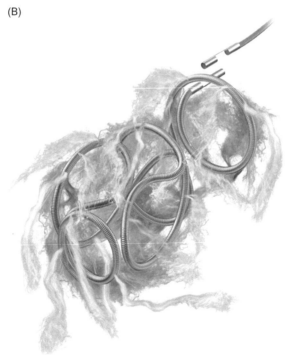

Figure 2.31 Example of a detachable coil that can be used for embolization in case of distal coronary perforation (Interlock, *Boston Scientific***).** (A) demonstrates deployment of the coil whereas (B) illustrates the coil configuration after delivery.

2.9.3   Pericardiocentesis Tray

Pericardiocentesis can be performed using a standard 0.018 needle, a J-tip 0.035 in. guidewire, and a standard pigtail catheter, however, having all equipment assembled in a premanufactured pericardiocentesis tray can facilitate and speed up the procedure.

2.10   Radiation Protection

Given that CTO procedures can be lengthy, it is ideal to minimize radiation exposure for both the patient and the operator, as described in detail in Chapter 10. There are several radiation protection pads that decrease radiation scatter from the patient, such as the RadPad (Worldwide Innovations & Technologies, Inc.) (Figure 2.32).

2.11   The "CTO cart"

Having a dedicated "CTO cart" (Figure 2.33) with all commonly used CTO PCI equipment (including equipment for managing complications, such as covered stents and coils) can facilitate and make CTO PCI more efficient.

In summary, there are many pieces of equipment that can be used in CTO PCI. Clearly, there is no "universal" CTO PCI equipment checklist and there is a great component of personal preference, experience, and availability in constructing a CTO checklist for each individual catheter laboratory and operator. Table 2.1 could serve as a starting point. Having the right tool for the right job can significantly simplify the procedure and boost success rates in CTO PCI.

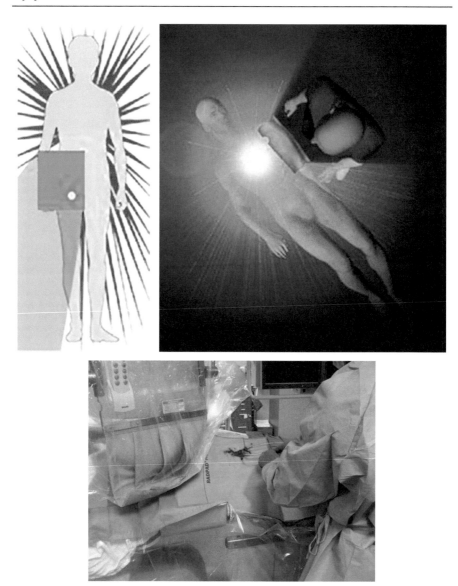

Figure 2.32 Illustration of use of radiation protection pads.
Source: Reproduced with permission from Worldwide Innovations &
Technologies, Inc.

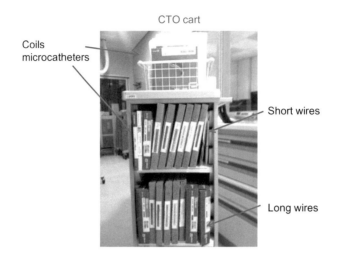

Figure 2.33 Example of a "CTO cart."

References

1. Brilakis ES. The essential equipment for CTO interventions. *Cardiol Today's Interv* 2013 [May June 2013].
2. Joyal D, Thompson CA, Grantham JA, Buller CEH, Rinfret S. The retrograde technique for recanalization of chronic total occlusions: a step-by-step approach. *JACC Cardiovasc Interv* 2012;**5**:1−11.
3. Brilakis ES, Grantham JA, Thompson CA, et al. The retrograde approach to coronary artery chronic total occlusions: a practical approach. *Catheter Cardiovasc Interv* 2012;**79**:3−19.
4. Brilakis ES, Grantham JA, Rinfret S, et al. A percutaneous treatment algorithm for crossing coronary chronic total occlusions. *JACC Cardiovasc Interv* 2012;**5**:367−79.
5. Wu EB, Chan WW, Yu CM. Retrograde chronic total occlusion intervention: tips and tricks. *Catheter Cardiovasc Interv* 2008;**72**:806−14.
6. Waksman MD, Saito S. *Chronic total occlusions: a guide to revascularization*. Wiley-Blackwell; 2013. Chapter 21. p. 149.
7. Tsuchikane E, Katoh O, Kimura M, Nasu K, Kinoshita Y, Suzuki T. The first clinical experience with a novel catheter for collateral channel tracking in retrograde approach for chronic coronary total occlusions. *JACC Cardiovasc Interv* 2010;**3**: 165−71.
8. McClure SJ, Wahr DW, Webb JG. Venture wire control catheter. *Catheter Cardiovasc Interv* 2005;**66**:346−50.

9. Naidu SS, Wong SC. Novel intracoronary steerable support catheter for complex coronary intervention. *J Invasive Cardiol* 2006;**18**:80−1.

10. McNulty E, Cohen J, Chou T, Shunk KA. "Grapple hook" technique using a deflectable tip catheter to facilitate complex proximal circumflex interventions. *Catheter Cardiovasc Interv* 2006;**67**:46−8.

11. Aranzulla TC, Colombo A, Sangiorgi GM. Successful endovascular renal artery aneurysm exclusion using the Venture catheter and covered stent implantation: a case report and review of the literature. *J Invasive Cardiol* 2007;**19**:E246−53.

12. Aranzulla TC, Sangiorgi GM, Bartorelli A, et al. Use of the Venture wire control catheter to access complex coronary lesions: how to turn procedural failure into success. *EuroIntervention* 2008;**4**:277−84.

13. Iturbe JM, Abdel-Karim AR, Raja VN, Rangan BV, Banerjee S, Brilakis ES. Use of the venture wire control catheter for the treatment of coronary artery chronic total occlusions. *Catheter Cardiovasc Interv* 2010;**76**:936−41.

14. Brilakis ES, Lombardi WL, Banerjee S. Use of the Stingray® Guidewire and the Venture® catheter for crossing flush coronary chronic total occlusions due to in-stent restenosis. *Catheter Cardiovasc Interv* 2010;**76**:391−4.

15. Werner GS. The BridgePoint devices to facilitate recanalization of chronic total coronary occlusions through controlled subintimal reentry. *Expert Rev Med Devices* 2011;**8**:23−9.

16. Brilakis ES, Lombardi WB, Banerjee S. Use of the Stingray guidewire and the Venture catheter for crossing flush coronary chronic total occlusions due to in-stent restenosis. *Catheter Cardiovasc Interv* 2010;**76**:391−4.

17. Brilakis ES, Badhey N, Banerjee S. "Bilateral knuckle" technique and Stingray re-entry system for retrograde chronic total occlusion intervention. *J Invasive Cardiol* 2011;**23**:E37−9.

18. Michael TT, Papayannis AC, Banerjee S, Brilakis ES. Subintimal dissection/reentry strategies in coronary chronic total occlusion interventions. *Circ Cardiovasc Interv* 2012;**5**:729−38.

19. Whitlow PL, Burke MN, Lombardi WL, et al. Use of a novel crossing and re-entry system in coronary chronic total occlusions that have failed standard crossing techniques: results of the FAST-CTOs (Facilitated Antegrade Steering Technique in Chronic Total Occlusions) trial. *JACC Cardiovasc Interv* 2012;**5**:393−401.

20. Papayannis A, Banerjee S, Brilakis ES. Use of the CrossBoss catheter in coronary chronic total occlusion due to in-stent restenosis. *Catheter Cardiovasc Interv* 2012;**80**:E30−6.

21. Fang HY, Lee CH, Fang CY, et al. Application of penetration device (Tornus) for percutaneous coronary intervention in balloon uncrossable chronic total occlusion-procedure outcomes, complications, and predictors of device success. *Catheter Cardiovasc Interv* 2011;**78**:356−62.
22. Papayannis AC, Michael TT, Brilakis ES. Challenges associated with use of the GuideLiner catheter in percutaneous coronary interventions. *J Invasive Cardiol* 2012;**24**: 370−1.
23. Luna M, Papayannis A, Holper EM, Banerjee S, Brilakis ES. Transfemoral use of the GuideLiner catheter in complex coronary and bypass graft interventions. *Catheter Cardiovasc Interv* 2012;**80**:437−46.
24. Mamas MA, Fath-Ordoubadi F, Fraser DG. Distal stent delivery with Guideliner catheter: first in man experience. *Catheter Cardiovasc Interv* 2010;**76**:102−11.
25. Romaguera R, Waksman R. Covered stents for coronary perforations: is there enough evidence? *Catheter Cardiovasc Interv* 2011;**78**: 246−53.
26. Brilakis ES, Karmpaliotis D, Patel V, Banerjee S. Complications of chronic total occlusion angioplasty. *Interv Cardiol Clin* 2012;**1**:373−89.
27. Ben-Gal Y, Weisz G, Collins MB, et al. Dual catheter technique for the treatment of severe coronary artery perforations. *Catheter Cardiovasc Interv* 2010;**75**:708−12.
28. Pershad A, Yarkoni A, Biglari D. Management of distal coronary perforations. *J Invasive Cardiol* 2008;**20**:E187−91.

3 The Basics: Timing, Dual Injection, Studying the Lesion, Access, Anticoagulation, Guide Support, Trapping

3.1 Timing

In general, CTO PCI should not be performed ad hoc in order to:[1]

> **a.** Allow time for thorough procedural planning and preparation, which is essential for success.
> **b.** Minimize the amount of contrast and radiation administered.
> **c.** Minimize patient and operator fatigue.
> **d.** Allow for a detailed discussion with the patient and family about the indications, goals, risks, and alternatives (such as medical therapy and coronary artery bypass graft surgery) to the procedure. Risks that may be increased in CTO PCI compared to non-CTO PCI include radiation injury and perforation.

In some cases, however, ad hoc PCI may be the best option, such as in patients who present with an acute coronary syndrome due to failure of a highly diseased saphenous vein graft, in whom treatment of the native coronary artery CTO is considered to be the preferred treatment strategy.[2]

Manual of Coronary Chronic Total Occlusion Interventions. DOI: http://dx.doi.org/10.1016/B978-0-12-420129-3.00003-9

3.2   Dual Injection

Dual injection angiography is of critical importance in CTO PCI. This is the simplest and most effective technique for increasing CTO PCI success rates and should be performed in all patients with contra-lateral collaterals.[3]

3.2.1   Why Is Dual Injection Key?

Dual injection provides the following benefits:[4]

Before PCI

a. Non-simultaneous, single catheter injection often provides suboptimal visualization of the CTO segment and limited ability to assess both the proximal and distal caps and the distal vessel beyond the CTO due to collateral competitive flow (Figures 3.1 and 3.2). Occasionally, dual injection will reveal that the "CTO" is not a total occlusion, but rather a "functional" occlusion with a central patent microchannel (Figure 3.1).

During PCI

a. Contralateral injection during CTO PCI allows **visualization of the guidewire position** during crossing attempts. If the guidewire is outside the vessel or in a side branch, it can be repositioned before advancing equipment, significantly reducing the risk of perforation or other complications (Figure 3.3).

b. Even if there are ipsilateral collaterals at baseline, during CTO PCI, the collateral flow direction and strength of flow can shift from one source to another due to ipsilateral collateral damage, not allowing determination of distal guidewire position.

c. When using dissection/re-entry techniques antegrade contrast injections may result in hydraulic enlargement of the subintimal space and reduce the chances of successful re-entry (Figure 3.4). We recommend removing the injecting syringe from the antegrade guide manifold during dissection/re-entry attempts to prevent inadvertent contrast injection and expansion of the subintimal space, as demonstrated in Figure 5.7.

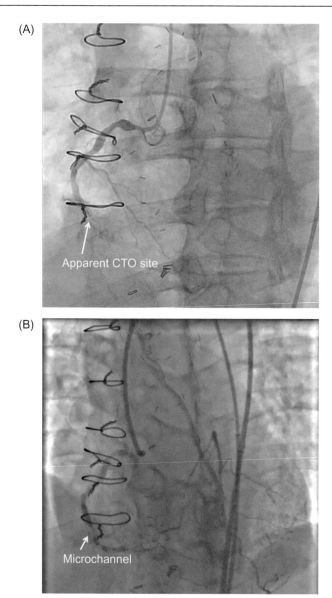

Figure 3.1 Example of dual injection revealing a "microchannel" at the assumed occlusion site. Injection of the right coronary artery revealed a distal right coronary artery occlusion (A), but the length of the occlusion and the quality of the distal vessel could not be determined. Dual injection (via the right coronary artery and the left internal mammary graft that supplied collaterals to the right posterior descending artery) demonstrated a microchannel at the occlusion site, very short "occlusion" length, and diffusely diseased distal vessel. Crossing of the CTO was easily achieved with a Fielder XT guidewire.

(A)

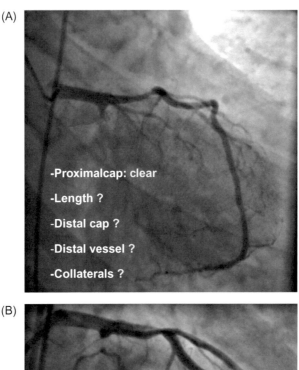

-Proximalcap: clear

-Length ?

-Distal cap ?

-Distal vessel ?

-Collaterals ?

(B)

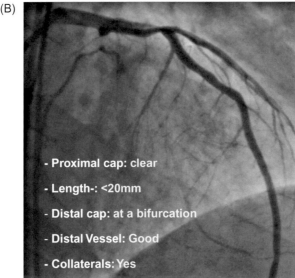

- Proximal cap: clear

- Length-: <20mm

- Distal cap: at a bifurcation

- Distal Vessel: Good

- Collaterals: Yes

Figure 3.2 Example of how dual injection can significantly improve the understanding of the CTO anatomy and CTO crossing options. Injection of the left main coronary artery demonstrates a proximal circumflex CTO (A), but the characteristics of the lesion remained unknown. Using dual injection (B), the characteristics of the CTO (proximal cap ambiguity, lesion length, bifurcation at distal cap, quality of distal vessel, and presence of collaterals) were clarified.
Source: Courtesy of Dr. Santiago Garcia.

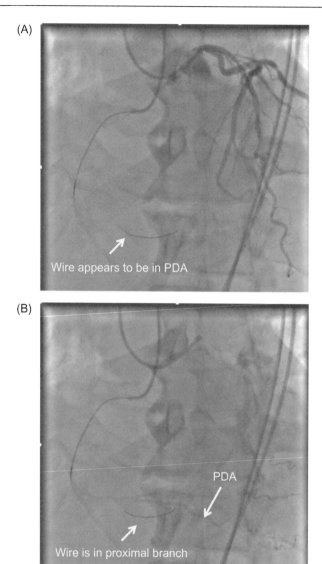

Figure 3.3 Dual injection to determine distal guidewire position after crossing. The guidewire appeared to be in the right posterior descending artery (PDA, A) but was actually in a proximal side branch (B). Dual injection allowed correction of guidewire position before balloon inflation and stent deployment. PDA = posterior descending artery.

(A)

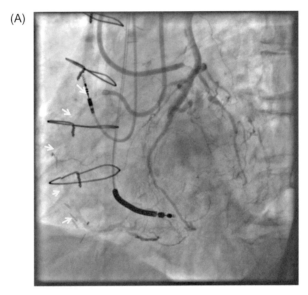

(B)

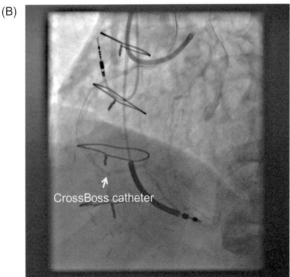

CrossBoss catheter

Figure 3.4 Contralateral injection for guiding stent placement after subintimal CTO crossing. A right coronary artery CTO (A) was subintimally crossed with the CrossBoss catheter (arrow, B), followed by re-entry using the Stingray balloon and a Pilot 200 wire ("stick and swap" technique, C and D). Contralateral injection was used to guide stent placement at the posterior descending artery/right posterolateral branch bifurcation (arrow, F) with an excellent final result (F).

(C)

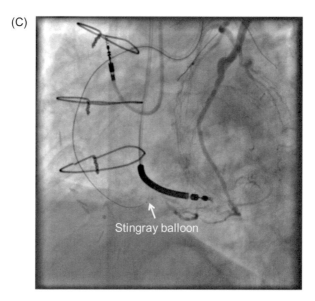

(D)

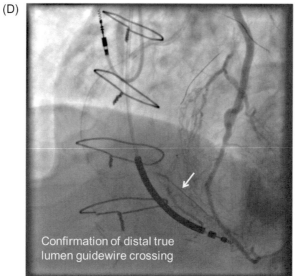

Figure 3.4 (Continued)

(E)

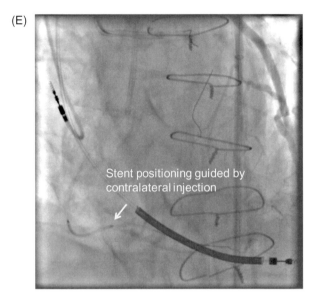

(F)

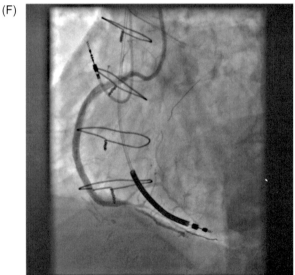

Figure 3.4 (Continued)

3.2.2 Dual Injection Technique

Dual injection should be performed as follows:

a. Introduce the right coronary artery guide catheter first (before inserting the left coronary artery guide catheter) to allow for unimpeded torqueing necessary to engage the right coronary artery ostium.

b. Use low magnification (13 in. instead of 8 in.) to enable visualization of the entire coronary circulation.

c. Do not pan the table to facilitate recognition of collaterals.

d. Obtain long cine acquisition to allow for the contrast to travel through the collateral vessels and fill the distal vessel.

e. Inject the donor vessel (vessel that supplies the territory distal to the CTO) first, followed by injection of the occluded vessel after collaterals have filled the distal vessel. To reduce radiation exposure, the donor vessel can be injected before cine is recorded.

A commonly employed method of allowing simultaneous injection of both coronaries **during the diagnostic angiogram without requiring a second point of access** is to upsize the femoral arterial access point to an 8-Fr sheath. Two 4 Fr catheters can then be passed through a single 8 Fr sheath to allow simultaneous injection of both coronaries.[5]

3.3 Studying the Lesion

3.3.1 How to Evaluate the Lesion?

Spending enough time to study the CTO angiographic parameters will make the procedure easier and will increase the likelihood of success. Any other previous angiograms should also be located and reviewed carefully.

By whom? Ideally the films should be reviewed by the entire CTO team, including the physicians, technicians, and fellows.

How long? Usually 15−30 min/patient.

Which parameters should be assessed?

There are four key parameters that should be evaluated during the angiographic review, as described in more detail in Chapter 7:[4]

1. Proximal cap ambiguity
2. Lesion length
3. Quality of distal target vessel
4. Collateral circulation

Assessment: Tips and Tricks

- Using slow replay and magnified views may help clarify the CTO vessel course and the collateral connections.
- Occasionally, tracing the collaterals backward may help identify their origin and course.
- In some patients pre-procedural coronary computed tomography may help decipher the course of the occluded vessel and evaluate the presence and extent of calcification. This is especially helpful in patients with very long occluded segments.

Why? To understand the CTO anatomy and collateral circulation, which enables the operator to map out all possible options for crossing the occlusion and create a strategic plan (Figure 3.5).

3.3.2   Collateral Evaluation

3.3.2.1   Collateral Classification Schemes

Collateral vessels can be assessed for:

a. Size (CC classification)
b. Tortuosity
c. Angle of connection.

Larger collaterals without tortuosity connecting to the distal vessel at an obtuse angle are the best for the retrograde approach. Examples of favorable and unfavorable collateral branches are shown in Figures 3.6 and 3.7.

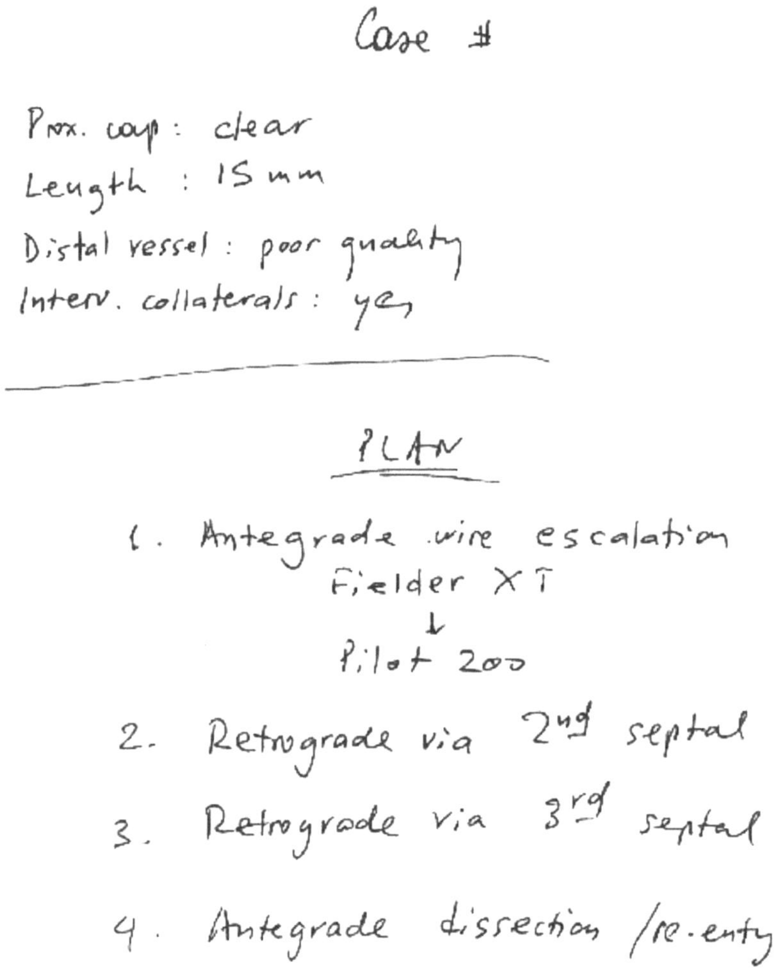

Case #

Prox. cap : clear
Length : 15 mm
Distal vessel : poor quality
Interv. collaterals : yes

PLAN

1. Antegrade wire escalation
   Fielder XT
   ↓
   Pilot 200

2. Retrograde via 2nd septal

3. Retrograde via 3rd septal

4. Antegrade dissection / re-entry

Figure 3.5 Example of a "strategic plan" for CTO PCI.

There are currently two collateral vessel classification systems (Table 3.1).

Note

The presence of collaterals does not necessarily signify viability of the collateralized myocardial territory, as collaterals can also develop to non-viable territories.[9]

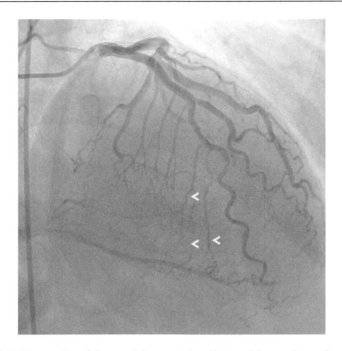

Figure 3.6 Example of favorable septal collateral branches. Septal collaterals (arrowheads) with continuous connection between the left anterior descending artery and the right posterior descending artery. *Source*: Modified with permission from Ref. 8.

3.3.2.2 Optimal Views for Visualizing Collaterals

1. Septal collaterals
   a. Right Anterior Oblique (RAO) cranial is best for determining the origin of the collateral.
   b. Straight RAO or RAO caudal is best for visualizing the part of the collateral closer to the posterior descending artery (PDA) which is usually more tortuous than the part that is closer to the left anterior descending artery (LAD).
   c. Left Anterior Oblique (LAO) view may be helpful during wiring attempts.
2. Epicardial collaterals in the lateral wall (diagonal-obtuse marginal vessels)
   a. LAO cranial
   b. RAO cranial
3. Epicardial collaterals between the proximal circumflex and RCA
   a. Anteroposterior (AP) caudal
   b. RAO

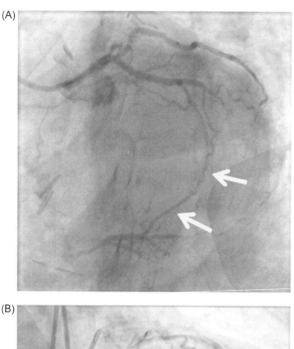

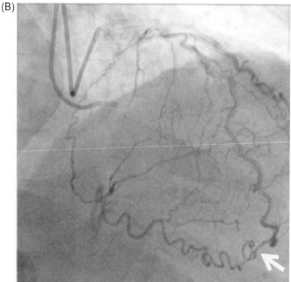

Figure 3.7 Examples of favorable and unfavorable epicardial collateral vessels.
(A) Favorable epicardial collateral from the circumflex to the right posterolateral branch with minimal tortuosity and adequate size.
(B) Unfavorable epicardial collateral from the left anterior descending artery to the right coronary artery with extreme tortuosity.
Source: Modified with permission from Ref. 8.

Table 3.1 Rentrop and Werner Classification of Coronary Collateral
Circulation

Rentrop classification[6] (developed for occluded and non-occluded arteries)	
0	No filling of collateral vessels
1	Filling of collateral vessels without any epicardial filling of the target artery
2	Partial epicardial filling by collateral vessels of the target artery
3	Complete epicardial filling by collateral vessels of the target artery (in CTOs, Rentrop 3 is prevalent in 85% of lesions)
Werner collateral connection grade[7]	
CC0	No continuous connection
CC1	Threadlike continuous connection
CC2	Side branch−like connection (≥0.4 mm)
CC3	>1 mm diameter of direct connection (not included in the original description)

3.3.3   Use of Computed Tomography

Although infrequently used at present, pre-procedural coronary computed tomography may provide assessment of calcification, tortuosity, and length of the occluded segment and also help to identify the
best angiographic projection for CTO crossing.[10] Occasionally, unex-
pected findings from computed tomography (such as prior stent
placed into a side branch—Figure 3.8) may significantly facilitate the
procedure.

3.4   Vascular Access

3.4.1   Dual Arterial Access

This is the most important step for increasing CTO PCI success rates
(see benefits of dual injection in Section 3.2). It should be used in all
cases, except the rare cases in which there are absolutely no contralateral collaterals.

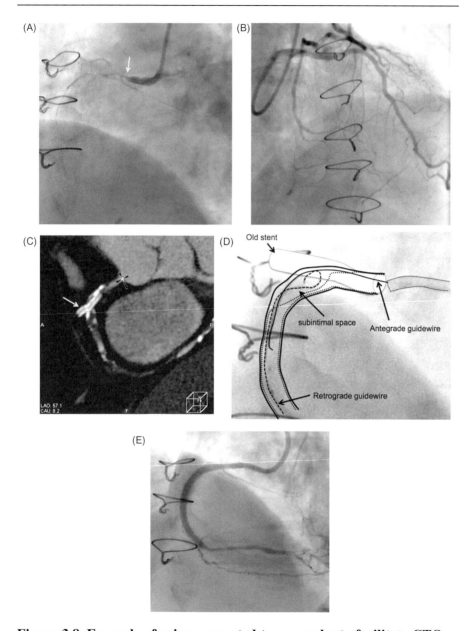

Figure 3.8 Example of using computed tomography to facilitate CTO PCI. Proximal right coronary artery CTO (arrow, A) with collateral filling of the right posterolateral branch from the LAD (B). CT angiography demonstrated that a prior stent (arrow, C) was actually placed into a side branch. The CTO was successfully crossed using the retrograde approach (D) with an excellent final result (E).

Source: Reproduced with permission from HMP Communications.[11]

> • Bifemoral access is preferred by most operators, especially early in the learning curve, as it may allow easier vessel engagement and enhanced guide catheter support (with use of large 8 Fr guide catheters); however, it carries increased risk of vascular access complications compared to the radial approach.
> • Femoral—radial access may be used, especially when the retrograde approach is unlikely to be utilized.
> • Biradial access can be successfully used in centers with significant radial access expertise (Section 2.1).[12]

Long femoral sheaths (usually 45 cm) enhance support and facilitate guide catheter manipulations.

3.4.2 "Advanced": Triple Arterial Access

Occasionally triple arterial access may be needed for CTO PCI. An example is a right coronary artery CTO with distal filling via the LAD, which is supplied by a LIMA (Figure 3.9), when a retrograde approach is planned via a septal collateral that originates proximal to the LAD occlusion.

3.5 Anticoagulation

• Unfractionated heparin is the preferred agent, because it can be reversed in case of severe perforation. The recommended activated clotting times (ACT) are:
  • > 300 s for antegrade CTO PCI.
  • > 350 s for retrograde CTO PCI (some operators use >300 s, but check ACT very frequently if it is in the low 300-s range).
• The ACT should be checked every 30 min.
• A small (4 Fr) femoral venous sheath can be inserted to facilitate ACT checking by the cath lab staff to minimize interruptions of the physician tasks.
• Bivalirudin is best avoided because its anticoagulant effect cannot be reversed. Moreover, there are unpublished cases in which guide thrombosis occurred during long procedures.

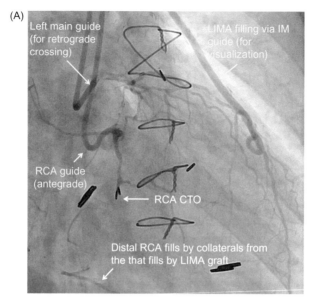

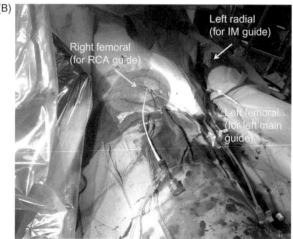

Figure 3.9 Example of triple arterial access. Bifemoral and left radial access was obtained to enable retrograde crossing of a right coronary artery CTO. The right femoral artery was used for engaging the right coronary artery, the left femoral artery for engaging the left main (through which retrograde crossing was performed), and the left radial artery for engaging the left internal mammary artery (through which visualization of the right posterior descending artery was achieved).
Source: Reproduced with permission from HMP Communications.[13]

- Glycoprotein IIb/IIIa inhibitors should NOT be given, **even after successful crossing and stenting** of the CTO, because a minor wire perforation could re-open and cause delayed pericardial effusion and tamponade.

3.6 Techniques to Increase Guide Catheter Support (Large Bore Guide, Active Guide Support, Guide Catheter Extensions, Anchor Techniques)

Strong guide support is essential for achieving high CTO PCI success rates and for maximizing efficiency, irrespective of the crossing technique selected. Techniques to increase guide catheter support include (Figure 3.10):

---

1. Deep guide catheter intubation (active support).[14]
2. Large and supportive shape guide catheters (passive support).
3. One or multiple buddy wires.[15]
4. Guide catheter extensions.
5. Anchor techniques.[16,17]

These techniques can also be used in combination: an example is the "Anchor−Tornus technique."[18]

3.6.1 Active Support

Deep guide catheter insertion can significantly increase backup support but carries a small risk of dissection. Active guide catheter support can be achieved by clockwise rotation for the right coronary artery and forward pushing for the left main (Figure 3.10B). It is important to be aware of the various guide tip characteristics from different manufacturers (softer versus sharper tips).

3.6.2 Passive Support

Passive guide support can be increased by larger size guides (Figure 3.10C) or more supportive shapes (such as Amplatz guide catheter, Figure 3.10D).

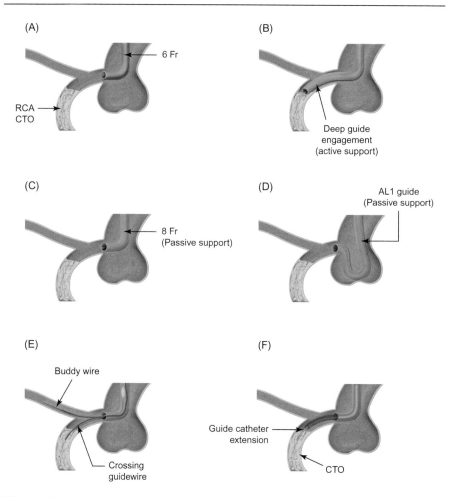

Figure 3.10 Overview of active and passive guide support techniques.

3.6.3   Buddy Wires

One or more buddy wires can be advanced in the main vessel or a side branch (Figure 3.10E), generally using supportive workhorse wires, a technique that usually provides only mild to moderate support.

3.6.4   Guide Catheter Extensions

Two guide catheter extensions are currently available in the United States: the Guideliner V2 catheter (Vascular Solutions) and the

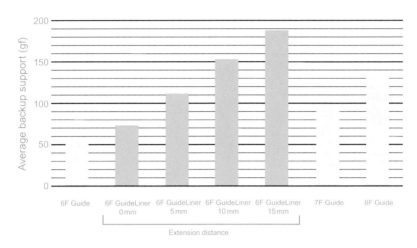

Figure 3.11 Illustration of the incremental guide catheter support achieved with use of the Guideliner catheter.
Source: Reproduced with permission from Vascular Solutions.

Guidezilla (Boston Scientific), which are described in detail in Section 2.7.2. Use of guide catheter extensions can significantly increase guide catheter support and allow use of smaller caliber guide catheters (Figures 3.10F and 3.11). A third guide catheter extension (Heartrail, Terumo, 5 Fr extension that fits through a 6-Fr guide catheter) is currently available outside the United States.

3.6.5 Anchor Techniques

Anchor techniques can be useful to increase guide catheter support. The most common is the **side-branch anchoring** technique, in which a balloon is inflated in a proximal side branch of the target vessel (Figure 3.12A).[18-27] In the **co-axial anchor** technique, a balloon is inflated in the coronary artery proximal to the occlusion, enhancing the guidewire penetration capacity (Figure 3.12B).[22] The **distal anchor** technique is similar to the side-branch anchor, except that the balloon is inflated distal to or at the occlusion within the target artery (Figures 3.12C and 3.13).[16,28] Two guidewires are required for the distal anchor technique, one to deliver the anchor balloon and a

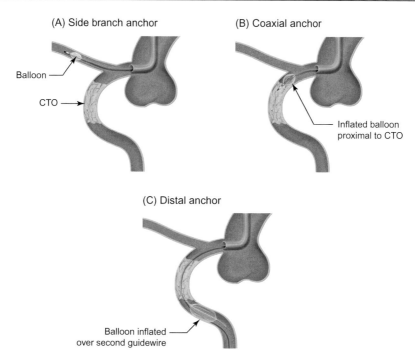

Figure 3.12 Illustration of the three anchor techniques.

second guidewire (which is pinned by the anchor balloon against the vessel wall), for delivering equipment, such as microcatheters, balloons, stents, and guide catheter extensions to the lesion (Figure 3.13).[21,23,29−31]

Limitations of the anchor techniques:

a. Injury at the site of the anchor balloon inflation, which is usually inconsequential in these small side branches.[16] The risk can be minimized by inflating the anchor balloon at relatively low pressures (6−8 atm).

b. Distal dissection can occur with the distal anchor technique, requiring extensive stenting.

c. Larger guide catheters (at least 7 Fr) are needed for delivering a distal anchor balloon and other equipment.[23,30,31]

d. Use of a side-branch anchor may modify the proximal vessel anatomy and hinder antegrade wiring.

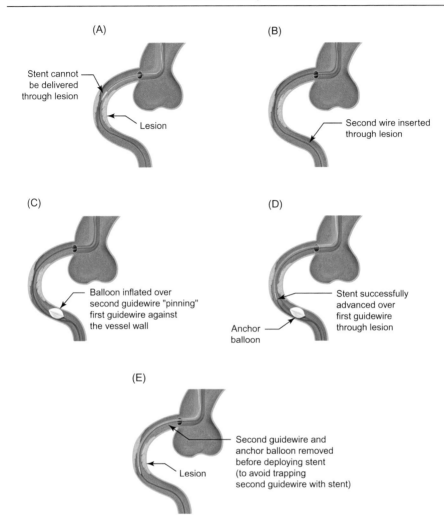

Figure 3.13 Step-by-step illustration of the distal anchor technique. The distal anchor technique can be useful when difficulty is encountered delivering a stent (or other equipment) through a lesion (A). A second guidewire is inserted next to the initial guidewire (B) and a balloon (which is usually easier to deliver than a stent) is delivered distal to the lesion and inflated, "pinning" the initial guidewire against the vessel wall (C) and enabling stent delivery over the first guidewire (D). The second guidewire (and balloon) are subsequently withdrawn before stent deployment (E).

3.7   Trapping

Trapping is the best technique for removing or exchanging micro-catheters or any over-the-wire system when using a short (180−190 cm) or even long (300 cm) guidewire (Figure 3.14A), because it:

a. Minimizes guidewire movement, which can result in guidewire position loss, distal vessel injury, and/or perforation.
b. Minimizes radiation exposure (as fluoroscopy is only needed during the initial phase of wire withdrawal).

The small inner diameter of a 6-Fr guide catheter prevents utilization of the trapping technique for over-the-wire balloons, the CrossBoss catheter, and the Stingray balloon. However, with a 6-Fr guide, trapping can be used to facilitate exchange of the Finecross and Corsair microcatheters because of the low profile of these devices.

3.7.1   Trapping Technique

Step 1: Withdraw the over-the-wire balloon and microcatheter into the guide catheter just proximal to the position where the trapping balloon will be inflated (Figure 3.14B).
Step 2: Insert the trapping balloon through the Y-connector, next to (but not over) the guidewire.
   Type of balloon: Rapid exchange, because over-the-wire balloons have higher profile and may not fit into the guide catheter along with other balloons, especially the Stingray balloon or the Venture catheter.
   Size of the balloon: 2.5 mm for 6 Fr; 3.0 mm for 7 and 8 Fr.
   Length: Ideally ≥ 20 mm (longer balloon length provides more area of contact and "pins" the wire better, which is especially important for trapping polymer-jacketed wires, which are more slippery).
   Caveats: A previously used trapping balloon may get deformed and be difficult to insert through the Y-connector on subsequent attempts. In such cases, the trapping balloon should be exchanged for a new one.
Step 3: Advance the trapping balloon to the distal portion of the guide catheter beyond the marker of the microcatheter or over-the-wire balloon, usually at or near the primary curve (Figure 3.14C).
   Caveat: When short guides are used, the balloon markers cannot be relied upon to prevent inadvertent advancement of the trapping balloon into the target vessel.

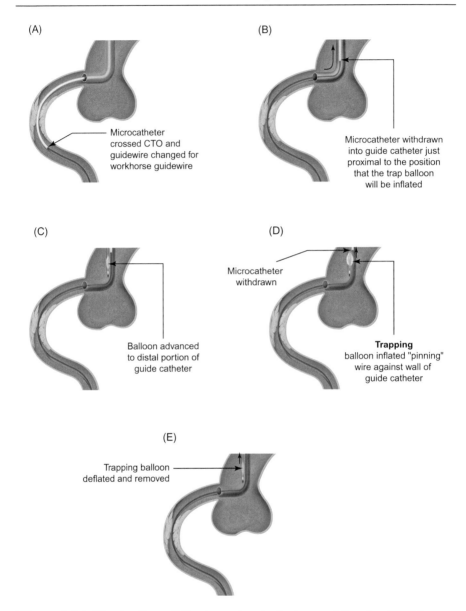

(A)

Microcatheter crossed CTO and guidewire changed for workhorse guidewire

(B)

Microcatheter withdrawn into guide catheter just proximal to the position that the trap balloon will be inflated

(C)

Balloon advanced to distal portion of guide catheter

(D)

Microcatheter withdrawn

Trapping balloon inflated "pinning" wire against wall of guide catheter

(E)

Trapping balloon deflated and removed

Figure 3.14 Illustration of the trapping technique. After the CTO has been crossed and the crossing guidewire replaced with a workhorse guidewire (A), the microcatheter (or over-the-wire balloon) is withdrawn into the guide catheter (B), the trapping balloon is advanced distal to the microcatheter tip (C) and inflated (D), enabling removal of the microcatheter. The trapping balloon is then deflated and removed.

Step 4: Inflate the trapping balloon (Figure 3.14D).

    Pressure: 15−20 atm to provide adequate "trapping."

    Caveat: Balloon may rupture if inflated next to "handmade" side holes.

Step 5: Withdraw the over-the-wire balloon and microcatheter from the guide catheter (Figure 3.14D). Once the trapping balloon is in place and inflated, fluoroscopy is generally not required to maintain distal wire position. Extra care must, however, be utilized when working with polymer-jacketed guidewires, as they have a tendency to slip past the inflated trap balloon if significant tension is exerted.

Step 6: Deflate and remove the trapping balloon (Figure 3.14E).

Step 7: Back bleed the Y-connector.

    This is a very important step, because often air is entrained into the guide catheter during trapping. If contrast is injected without back bleeding, coronary air embolization is likely to occur.

Step 8: The microcatheter has been successfully removed while maintaining distal wire position.

In summary, knowledge and consistent application of the following seven "basic" techniques can significantly enhance the likelihood of CTO PCI success:

1. Avoiding ad hoc procedures.
2. Performing dual injection in nearly all cases.
3. Carefully studying the target lesion before the procedure.
4. Using long, bifemoral, 8 Fr arterial sheaths.
5. Optimizing anticoagulation.
6. Applying various techniques to increase guide catheter support.
7. Consistently using the trapping technique for equipment exchanges.

References

1. Blankenship JC, Gigliotti OS, Feldman DN, et al. Ad hoc percutaneous coronary intervention: a consensus statement from the Society for Cardiovascular Angiography and Interventions. *Catheter Cardiovasc Interv* 2013;**81**:748−58.
2. Brilakis ES, Banerjee S, Lombardi WL. Retrograde recanalization of native coronary artery chronic occlusions via acutely occluded vein grafts. *Catheter Cardiovasc Interv* 2010;**75**:109−13.

3. Singh M, Bell MR, Berger PB, Holmes Jr. DR. Utility of bilateral coronary injections during complex coronary angioplasty. *J Invasive Cardiol* 1999;**11**:70−4.

4. Brilakis ES, Grantham JA, Rinfret S, et al. A percutaneous treatment algorithm for crossing coronary chronic total occlusions. *JACC Cardiovasc Interv* 2012;**5**:367−79.

5. Nicholson WJ, Rab T. Simultaneous diagnostic coronary angiography utilizing a single arterial access technique. *Catheter Cardiovasc Interv* 2006;**68**:718.

6. Rentrop KP, Cohen M, Blanke H, Phillips RA. Changes in collateral channel filling immediately after controlled coronary artery occlusion by an angioplasty balloon in human subjects. *J Am Coll Cardiol* 1985;**5**:587−92.

7. Werner GS, Ferrari M, Heinke S, et al. Angiographic assessment of collateral connections in comparison with invasively determined collateral function in chronic coronary occlusions. *Circulation* 2003;**107**:1972−7.

8. Joyal D, Thompson CA, Grantham JA, Buller CEH, Rinfret S. The retrograde technique for recanalization of chronic total occlusions: a step-by-step approach. *JACC Cardiovasc Interv* 2012;**5**:1−11.

9. Heil M, Schaper W. Influence of mechanical, cellular, and molecular factors on collateral artery growth (arteriogenesis). *Circ Res* 2004;**95**:449−58.

10. Magro M, Schultz C, Simsek C, et al. Computed tomography as a tool for percutaneous coronary intervention of chronic total occlusions. *EuroIntervention* 2010;**6**(Suppl. G):G123−31.

11. Takimura H, Muramatsu T, Tsukahara R. CT coronary angiography-guided percutaneous coronary intervention for chronic total occlusion combined with retrograde approach. *J Invasive Cardiol* 2012;**24**:E5−9.

12. Burzotta F, De Vita M, Lefevre T, Tommasino A, Louvard Y, Trani C. Radial approach for percutaneous coronary interventions on chronic total occlusions: technical issues and data review. *Catheter Cardiovasc Interv* 2013. [published online before print].

13. Michael TT, Banerjee S, Brilakis ES. Role of internal mammary artery bypass grafts in retrograde chronic total occlusion interventions. *J Invasive Cardiol* 2012;**24**:359−62.

14. Von Sohsten R, Oz R, Marone G, McCormick DJ. Deep intubation of 6 French guiding catheters for transradial coronary interventions. *J Invasive Cardiol* 1998;**10**:198−202.

15. Burzotta F, Trani C, Mazzari MA, et al. Use of a second buddy wire during percutaneous coronary interventions: a simple solution for some challenging situations. *J Invasive Cardiol* 2005;**17**:171−4.

16. Di Mario C, Ramasami N. Techniques to enhance guide catheter support. *Catheter Cardiovasc Interv* 2008;**72**:505–12.

17. Saeed B, Banerjee S, Brilakis ES. Percutaneous coronary intervention in tortuous coronary arteries: associated complications and strategies to improve success. *J Interv Cardiol* 2008;**21**:504–11.

18. Kirtane AJ, Stone GW. The Anchor-Tornus technique: a novel approach to "uncrossable" chronic total occlusions. *Catheter Cardiovasc Interv* 2007;**70**:554–7.

19. Fujita S, Tamai H, Kyo E, et al. New technique for superior guiding catheter support during advancement of a balloon in coronary angioplasty: the anchor technique. *Catheter Cardiovasc Interv* 2003;**59**:482–8.

20. Hirokami M, Saito S, Muto H. Anchoring technique to improve guiding catheter support in coronary angioplasty of chronic total occlusions. *Catheter Cardiovasc Interv* 2006;**67**:366–71.

21. Matsumi J, Saito S. Progress in the retrograde approach for chronic total coronary artery occlusion: a case with successful angioplasty using CART and reverse-anchoring techniques 3 years after failed PCI via a retrograde approach. *Catheter Cardiovasc Interv* 2008;**71**:810–4.

22. Fang HY, Wu CC, Wu CJ. Successful transradial antegrade coronary intervention of a rare right coronary artery high anterior downward takeoff anomalous chronic total occlusion by double-anchoring technique and retrograde guidance. *Int Heart J* 2009;**50**:531–8.

23. Lee NH, Suh J, Seo HS. Double anchoring balloon technique for recanalization of coronary chronic total occlusion by retrograde approach. *Catheter Cardiovasc Interv* 2009;**73**:791–4.

24. Saito S. Different strategies of retrograde approach in coronary angioplasty for chronic total occlusion. *Catheter Cardiovasc Interv* 2008;**71**:8–19.

25. Surmely JF, Katoh O, Tsuchikane E, Nasu K, Suzuki T. Coronary septal collaterals as an access for the retrograde approach in the percutaneous treatment of coronary chronic total occlusions. *Catheter Cardiovasc Interv* 2007;**69**:826–32.

26. Surmely JF, Tsuchikane E, Katoh O, et al. New concept for CTO recanalization using controlled antegrade and retrograde subintimal tracking: the CART technique. *J Invasive Cardiol* 2006;**18**:334–8.

27. Rathore S, Katoh O, Matsuo H, et al. Retrograde percutaneous recanalization of chronic total occlusion of the coronary arteries: procedural outcomes and predictors of success in contemporary practice. *Circ Cardiovasc Interv* 2009;**2**:124–32.

28. Mahmood A, Banerjee S, Brilakis ES. Applications of the distal anchoring technique in coronary and peripheral interventions. *J Invasive Cardiol* 2011;**23**:291−4.
29. Christ G, Glogar D. Successful recanalization of a chronic occluded left anterior descending coronary artery with a modification of the retrograde proximal true lumen puncture technique: the antegrade microcatheter probing technique. *Catheter Cardiovasc Interv* 2009;**73**:272−5.
30. Mamas MA, Fath-Ordoubadi F, Fraser DG. Distal stent delivery with Guideliner catheter: first in man experience. *Catheter Cardiovasc Interv* 2010;**76**:102−11.
31. Fang HY, Fang CY, Hussein H, et al. Can a penetration catheter (Tornus) substitute traditional rotational atherectomy for recanalizing chronic total occlusions? *Int Heart J* 2010;**51**:147−52.

4 Antegrade Wire Escalation: The Foundation of CTO PCI

Antegrade wire escalation is the simplest and most widely used CTO crossing technique.[1−3] Familiarity and confidence with this technique provides the foundation upon which all other CTO PCI techniques (antegrade dissection/re-entry and retrograde) are built. Wire escalation is most appropriate for short occlusions, i.e., <20 mm length, longer occlusions where a through-and-through microchannel is suspected and in selected cases of occlusive in-stent restenosis.

Step 1 Selecting a Microcatheter or Over-the-Wire Balloon for Guidewire Support

Goal
Select the equipment most likely to assist with CTO crossing.

A microcatheter or over-the-wire balloon should be used for antegrade crossing in all CTOs (i.e., CTO crossing *should not* be attempted with unsupported guidewires).

A microcatheter is preferred by most operators (as described in Section 2.3), because it:

a. Enhances the wire-penetrating capacity.
b. Allows wire tip reshaping without losing wire position.
c. Facilitates wire exchanges.
d. Allows accurate assessment of the microcatheter tip location (because the marker is located at the tip, whereas in 1.20−1.50 mm balloons the marker is located in mid shaft and the tip is not angiographically visible).

These advantages are particularly important in cases of **tortuosity**, because over-the-wire balloons:

a. Are prone to kinking upon wire removal, thus hindering reliable wire exchanges.[4]
b. Are more likely to cause proximal vessel injury.[4]

Manual of Coronary Chronic Total Occlusion Interventions. DOI: http://dx.doi.org/10.1016/B978-0-12-420129-3.00004-0

Step 2 Getting to the CTO

Goal
Deliver a guidewire and microcatheter/over-the-wire balloon to the proximal CTO cap.

How?
Unless the CTO proximal cap is ostial or very proximal, it should be accessed with a workhorse guidewire advanced through a microcatheter, an over-the-wire balloon, or the CrossBoss catheter.

CTO wires with high penetrating power and tapered tips should not be used to traverse the proximal vessel to get to the CTO segment because:

a. They can cause vessel injury, especially in diffusely diseased vessels (Figure 4.1).

b. The wire bend required to reach the CTO is usually different (much larger) than the wire bend used when entering and crossing the CTO (much smaller) (Figure 4.2).

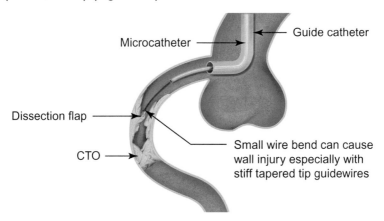

Figure 4.1 Illustration of proximal vessel injury during attempts to reach the proximal CTO cap.

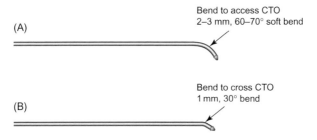

Figure 4.2 Example of guidewire bends used to reach the CTO (A) and traverse a CTO (B).

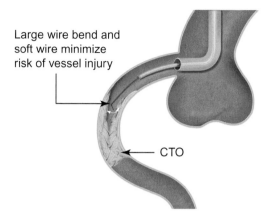

Figure 4.3 Reaching the CTO proximal cap using a soft-tipped guidewire.

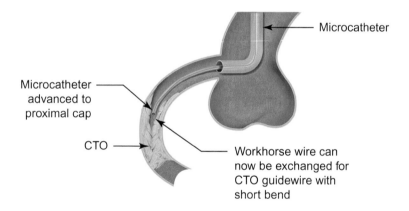

Figure 4.4 Exchange of the workhorse guidewire for a CTO crossing guidewire with a short tip.

A soft-tipped, workhorse guidewire should be used to reach the CTO proximal cap, followed by the microcatheter or over-the-wire balloon (Figure 4.3). The guidewire is then switched for the CTO crossing guidewire through the microcatheter or over-the-wire balloon (Figure 4.4).

Pearl of Wisdom

The best way to prolong (or fail) a case is by taking shortcuts!
Success is not the result of big actions; instead it is the results of small steps taken carefully!

Step 3 Selecting a Guidewire for CTO Crossing

Goal
Select the most appropriate guidewire for initial antegrade CTO crossing.

How?
Although several coronary guidewires are available for CTO crossing, a simplified selection and escalation scheme is currently preferred (Figure 4.5).[4]

A detailed description of the guidewires and their properties is presented in Section 2.4. A tapered, polymer-jacketed wire (such as the Fielder XT) is usually used first to track a microchannel (which may sometimes be invisible). This attempt should be brief, unless progress is achieved.

If this wire fails to cross, and the course of the CTO vessel is well understood (especially if the CTO is short), a stiff, tapered guidewire (such as Confianza Pro 12) is preferred. If the course of the CTO is unclear, then a stiff, polymer-jacketed guidewire (such as the Pilot 200) is preferred, because it is more likely to "track" the vessel architecture than exit the vessel wall.

If the proximal cap is heavily calcified, then a Confianza Pro 12 guidewire may need to be used initially to puncture the proximal cap and enable guidewire entrance into the occlusion.

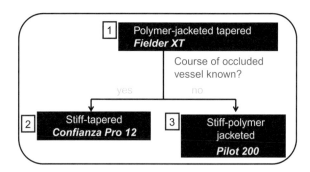

Figure 4.5 Illustration of guidewire escalation during antegrade CTO crossing attempts.

Step 4 Guidewire Tip Shaping

Goal
Shape the wire tip to maximize the likelihood of successful CTO crossing.

How?
A small (1 mm long, 30—45°) distal bend (Figure 4.6, panel A) is preferred for CTO crossing because it:

a. Enhances the penetrating capacity of the guidewire.
b. Facilitates entry into microchannels.
c. Reduces the likelihood of early deflection outside the vessel architecture or into branches arising within the occlusion.

Creating such a small bend can only be accomplished by inserting the guidewire through an introducer, rather than using the side of the introducer, as is commonly done for workhorse guidewires (Figure 4.7).

a. The guidewire is inserted through an introducer with approximately 1 mm protruding through the tip.
b. The guidewire tip is bent by 30—45° (sometimes a syringe is used to bend the tip of very stiff guidewires, such as the Confianza Pro 12 guidewire, as they can puncture the operator's glove).
c. The guidewire tip is inspected to verify optimal shaping.

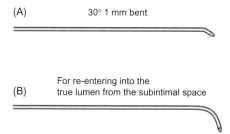

(A)   30° 1 mm bent

(B)   For re-entering into the
true lumen from the subintimal space

Figure 4.6 Illustration of wire tip bends for proximal cap penetration (A) and re-entering into the true lumen from the subintimal space (B).

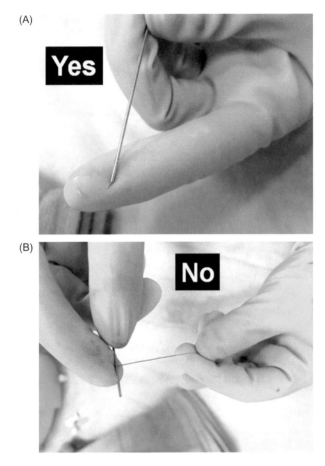

Figure 4.7 How to shape a guidewire for CTO intervention. (A) How to shape a wire (by inserting it through an introducer). (B) What to avoid in CTO wire shaping (i.e., using side of introducer).

d. The guidewire is withdrawn into the introducer and advanced into the microcatheter or over-the-wire balloon (it is best to insert the shaped guidewires into a microcatheter using an introducer to prevent potential tip damage or deformation).

Step 5 Advancing the Guidewire: Sliding Versus Drilling Versus Penetration

Goal
Cross CTO into the distal true lumen.

How?

Traditionally, three guidewire handling techniques have been described, two (sliding and drilling) used for both non-CTO and CTO lesions, and one (penetration) used for CTO lesions. Combinations of these techniques are often used, as part of the simplified wire escalation algorithm shown in Figure 4.5.

1. **Sliding** is usually the first step in CTO crossing and consists of forward movement of a tapered, polymer-jacketed guidewire, aiming to track microchannels within the CTO. The wire is advanced with gentle tip rotation and probing, i.e., a modest controlled drilling movement. These wires provide limited tactile feedback; hence, visual assessment of the wire course is important. If the wire fails to progress within a few minutes, change of guidewire and advancement technique is performed.
2. **Drilling** consists of controlled rotation of the guidewire in both directions. Rotation should be limited to <90° in each direction. Usually guidewires with moderate tip stiffness (3–6 g) are used, followed by escalation to stiffer wires (stiffer wires provide less tactile feedback). A small tip bend is crucial for this technique to avoid the creation of a large subintimal space.
3. **Penetration** consists of forward guidewire advancement intentionally steering (directing) the wire, not blindly rotating it, usually using a stiff (such as Miracle 12 or Confianza Pro 12) guidewire. The guidewire is used as a "needle" to penetrate the occlusion. This technique is important for lesions with a calcified, hard-to-penetrate, proximal cap and for steering though shorter occlusions when the vessel course is well understood.

Wire Advancement: Tips and Tricks

1. A microcatheter or over-the-wire balloon should be used to support the guidewire during crossing attempts to enhance the penetrating capacity of the guidewire (Section 2.3) and to allow for easy guidewire reshaping and exchanges.
2. Flexibility is important: if no progress is achieved within a few minutes, the wire and wire advancement strategy is modified.
3. Alternating between approximately orthogonal views frequently prevents inadvertent departure from the intended guidewire course, especially when directed penetration is employed. Vessel wall calcifications can also be very helpful as an aid for determining the vessel course and guidewire location.

Step 6 Assess Wire Position

Goal
Determine the guidewire position after crossing attempts. It is critical to understand the guidewire course *before* proceeding with microcatheter or balloon advancement to prevent perforation.

How?
There are three possible outcomes after the guidewire advances through the lesion:

a. Crossing into the distal true lumen.
b. Crossing into the subintimal space.
c. Exiting the vessel "architecture" (wire perforation).

How can the guidewire location be ascertained?

1. *Contralateral injection*: This is the best method when collaterals arise primarily from the contralateral coronary artery. Two orthogonal views are pivotally important, except in very straightforward cases.
2. Sudden, spontaneous freedom of the wire tip or proximal end movement as one passes the distal cap gives an important clue that distal true lumen wire position has been achieved. When moved forcefully or spun, however, stiff wires will create sufficient subintimal space to simulate a true lumen position.
3. *Distal wiring with a workhorse guidewire*: A microcatheter is advanced over the CTO crossing guidewire, which is exchanged for a workhorse guidewire. Easy advancement of a workhorse wire, especially if branches can be intentionally selected, indicates a true lumen position.
4. Two other methods can be used, but both are suboptimal and both require that the operator is certain (based on dual injection), that the guidewire is NOT outside the vessel architecture:

   • Intravascular ultrasound: However, advancing the IVUS catheter into the subintimal space can extend the dissection and hinder wire re-entry attempts.
   • Contrast injection through the microcatheter or over-the-wire balloon: This maneuver will cause staining if the microcatheter is located into the subintimal space, hence its use is NOT recommended.

> ### Assessing Wire Position: Tips and Tricks
> During CTO crossing, equipment should NEVER be advanced over a guidewire if the wire is suspected to be outside the vessel "architecture" based upon careful angiography or the wire's behavior. Otherwise, severe coronary perforation can occur.

Step 7a Wire Crosses into the Distal True Lumen
Goal
Complete CTO PCI with balloon and stents.

How?

1. Advance the microcatheter/over-the-wire balloon into the distal true lumen. Additional measures such as balloon anchoring in proximal side branches may be required to assist crossing of the CTO with a micro-catheter or over-the-wire balloon, as described in Chapter 8.
2. Remove the CTO crossing guidewire and exchange it for a workhorse guidewire.
3. Remove the microcatheter (ideally using the trapping technique to minimize wire motion and use of fluoroscopy, as described in Section 3.7).
4. Proceed with standard balloon angioplasty and stenting.

Step 7b Wire Enters the Subintimal Space
Goal
Enter into the distal true lumen.

How?
If the guidewire is found to be in the subintimal space when advanced past the distal cap, the following techniques can be used:

a. Bring a microcatheter into the subintimal space and position its tip adjacent to a well-seen segment of distal true lumen. In a projection that provides for good navigation, use directed penetration to re-enter the lumen. Avoid extending the subintimal track in an uncontrolled fashion.

b. Subintimal crossing and re-entry techniques (described in Chapter 5).

A knuckle wire or dissection catheter (i.e., the CrossBoss catheter) can be used to subintimally cross all the way to the distal true lumen, followed by wire-based or device-based (i.e., Stingray-based) re-entry attempts. A CrossBoss catheter can extend the subintimal track in a controlled fashion that minimizes the risk for hematoma formation.

Or

c. Use other techniques (currently not favored by many "hybrid" operators, as described in Chapter 7):

- Parallel wire
- See-saw
- Dual lumen microcatheter for redirection.

The above three techniques are based on the assumption that the original guidewire will prevent entry of additional guidewires into the

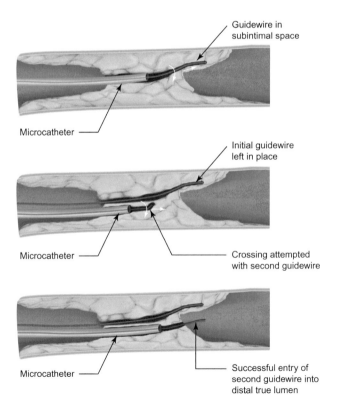

Figure 4.8 Illustration of the parallel-wire technique.

subintimal space. In all these techniques, the initial guidewire is left in place and crossing is attempted with a second guidewire that is advanced next to the original guidewire, either through a second microcatheter (see-saw technique), or without a second microcatheter (parallel-wire technique), or through a dual lumen catheter.

Parallel-wire and see-saw techniques

The parallel-wire technique is one of the oldest and most popular techniques for CTO PCI,[5,6] although it has recently decreased in popularity among "hybrid" operators in favor of subintimal dissection/re-entry techniques.

In the parallel-wire technique (Figure 4.8), when the guidewire enters the subintimal space (or occasionally a side branch), it is left in place, and a second guidewire is advanced "parallel" to the first wire until it enters into the distal true lumen. In the parallel-wire technique, a support catheter is used only for one guidewire, whereas in a variation of the parallel-wire technique called the "see-saw" technique (Figure 4.9) two microcatheters (or over-the-wire balloons) are used to support both

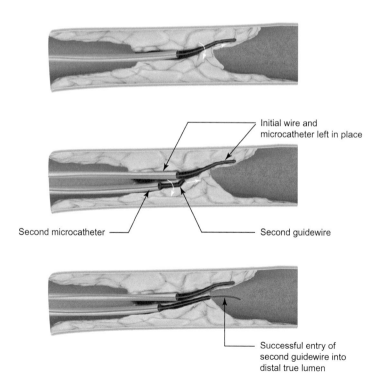

Figure 4.9 Illustration of the "see-saw" technique.

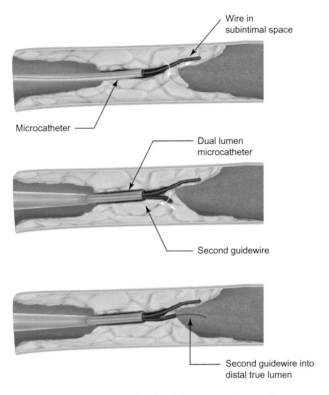

Figure 4.10 Illustration of use of a dual lumen catheter for achieving distal true lumen entry during antegrade crossing attempts once the first guidewire enters the subintimal space.

guidewires. Alternatively, a dual lumen microcatheter, such as the Twin-Pass (Vascular Solutions) or the Crusade (Kaneka Corp., Tokyo, Japan—not available in the United States at present) can be used to direct the second guidewire (Figure 4.10).[7]

Parallel-Wire Technique: Tips and Tricks

1. Prolonged parallel-wire attempts can cause enlargement of the sub-intimal space and hinder re-entry attempts. As a result parallel-wire strategies are not currently favored among "hybrid" operators (who prefer to proceed directly to re-entry using a dedicated re-entry system, as described in Chapter 5).

2. Use of two microcatheters (see-saw technique) is advantageous, as it allows better support and easier reshaping of the second guidewire.
3. Use of contrast and fluoroscopy may be decreased with parallel-wire techniques, as the first guidewire acts as a "marker" that guides advancement of the second guidewire.
4. The wires most commonly used as second "parallel" guidewires are stiff and highly torqueable wires, such as the Confianza Pro 12 and Miracle 12, or stiff polymer-jacketed guidewires, such as the Pilot 200.
5. Rotation of the second guidewire should be limited (i.e., the wire should not be "spinned") to minimize the likelihood of wrapping around the first guidewire.
6. Although leaving the first guidewire in place may block entrance of the second guidewire into the same space, occasionally the second guidewire may follow the path of the first guidewire; hence, early redirection of the guidewire within the CTO is important to create a new pathway.
7. It may sometimes be difficult to adequately visualize both guidewires, but this can be facilitated by the use of orthogonal angiographic views, which also allows understanding of the exact guidewire position during advancement.
8. Occasionally >2 guidewires can be used in parallel-wire techniques, but wire visualization can be very challenging due to overlap.
9. Sometimes the tip of the second guidewire may require a more acute bend to find the distal true lumen.

Step 7c Wire Outside the Vessel "Architecture"

If the guidewire exits the vessel "architecture" (vessel's adventitia), it should be withdrawn, followed by repeat crossing attempts using the same or a different guidewire. Wire exit without advancing a microcatheter or other equipment is very unlikely to cause perforation or tamponade due to the small caliber of the guidewire.

Occasionally the guidewire may enter a side branch and appear as if it has exited the vessel architecture. Therefore, careful assessment of the diagnostic angiogram is critical for understanding the coronary anatomy and guidewire position.

4.1   Special Situations

4.1.1   Proximal Cap Ambiguity

If the location of the proximal cap remains ambiguous (such as in flush or aortoostial occlusions), after detailed coronary angiography using dual injections, a primary retrograde approach is favored, if "interventional" collaterals are present. However, apparent cap ambiguity can sometimes be overcome, especially when the diagnostic images were obtained without the explicit intent to treat the CTO.

How can proximal cap ambiguity be clarified?

1. Repeat angiography with multiple, tightly coned and magnified projections to determine whether a "nub" or entry point into the CTO is present.
2. Perform IVUS guided puncture (Figure 4.11).
3. Do coronary computed tomography angiography (CTA) to clarify the proximal cap and vessel anatomy.

4.1.2   Bifurcation at Proximal Cap

In lesions with a side branch adjacent to the CTO, the antegrade wire may slide into the side branch and fail to engage the CTO (Figure 4.12A).

There are several techniques to successfully cross such lesions:

1. Insertion of a second guidewire into the side branch, which can act as a marker of the side-branch origin, facilitating antegrade crossing attempts with a second guidewire. In addition, the second wire can help protect larger side branches should the ostium of the side branch get compromised/dissected during aggressive CTO wiring of the proximal cap. Insertion of a stiff guidewire and/or balloon inflation in the side branch can induce a geometrical shift of the hard plaque and enable guidewire entry into the CTO (this has been called the "**open-sesame**" technique).[8]
2. *"Deflecting balloon"*: A balloon is inflated at the ostium of the side branch, "blocking" entry of the guidewire into the side branch, which can then engage the CTO proximal cap (Figure 4.12B).
3. Use of a dual lumen microcatheter (such as the Twin-Pass or Crusade catheters) to direct the second wire into the CTO proximal cap.[7]
4. Use of a wire directing catheter, such as the Venture catheter (Figure 4.13).[9]

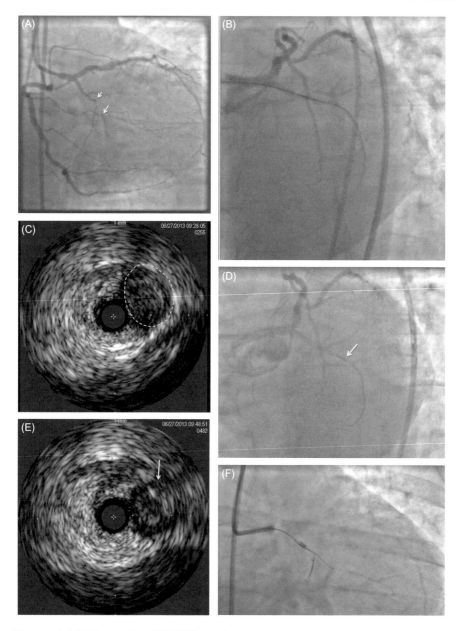

Figure 4.11 Example of IVUS used to resolve proximal cap ambiguity.
Ostial CTO of the first obtuse marginal branch (arrows, A). Repeat antegrade
crossing attempts were unsuccessful and the guidewire frequently entered the
distal circumflex (B). IVUS demonstrated that the CTO (yellow circle, C)
actually originated proximal (arrow, D) to the distal circumflex apparent
origin. During repeat antegrade crossing attempts a Confianza Pro 12

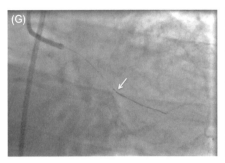
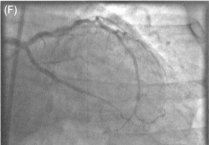

Figure 4.11 (Continued)

4.1.3 Bifurcation at Distal Cap

When there is a bifurcation at the CTO distal cap (Figure 4.14A), the antegrade wire may cross into one of the branches (Figure 4.14B), whereas wiring of the other branch may be challenging.

Prolonged antegrade wiring attempts with a second guidewire may cause dissection of the other branch ostium and side-branch occlusion. In such cases, the "hairpin-wire" (also called *reversed guidewire*[10,11]) technique can be useful in directing a guidewire from the side branch into the main vessel.[12] In this technique, a polymer-jacketed wire is bent approximately 3 cm from the wire tip (Figure 4.15), advanced into the side branch (Figure 4.14C), and pulled back (Figure 4.14D) entering the main branch (Figure 4.14E).

What can go wrong?

Use of the "hairpin-wire" technique may cause vessel dissection. Also after the "hairpin" enters the main vessel, further advancement may be challenging due to the bend in the wire.

4.1.4 Ostial Circumflex CTO

Ostial circumflex CTOs may be challenging to cross due to angulation: Use of the Venture catheter can help direct and support the wire to cross the lesion (Figure 4.16).

◂ guidewire was utilized and its location within the CTO was confirmed by IVUS (arrow, E) before advancing it through the occlusion (F). Due to subintimal crossing the Stingray balloon and wire were used for re-entry (arrow, G) with a successful final outcome (H).

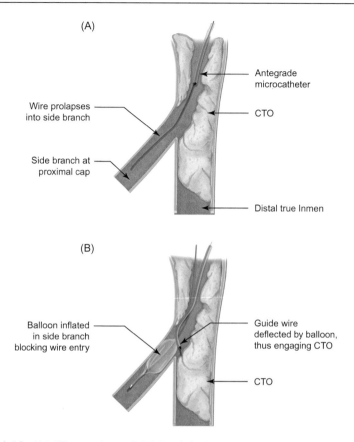

(A)

Antegrade microcatheter

Wire prolapses into side branch

CTO

Side branch at proximal cap

Distal true lnmen

(B)

Balloon inflated in side branch blocking wire entry

Guide wire deflected by balloon, thus engaging CTO

CTO

Figure 4.12 (A) Illustration of CTO with side branch originating adjacent to the proximal cap. (B) Illustration of the "deflecting balloon" technique for crossing CTOs with a side branch originating at the proximal cap.

4.1.5 In-Stent Restenosis CTOs

CTOs due to in-stent occlusion represent 5−25% of the total CTO intervention case volume and can be challenging,[13−17] especially in the presence of a large side branch in LAD occlusions or in the presence of tortuosity in RCA lesions.[18,19] It is ideal to prevent wire exit behind the stent, as that would lead to "crushing" of the restenosed stent after additional stent implantation.

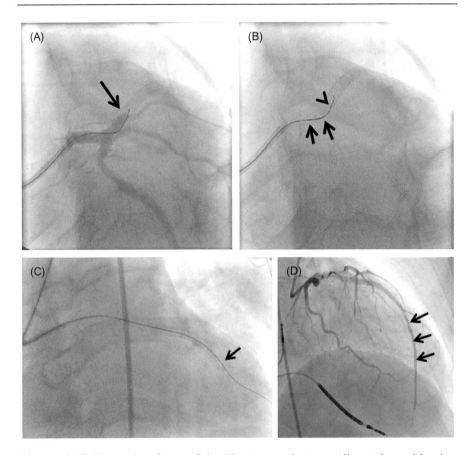

Figure 4.13 Example of use of the Venture catheter to direct the guidewire away from a side branch arising at the CTO proximal cap.
Source: Modified with permission from Ref. 9.

Potential crossing options include:

a. Antegrade wire escalation.
b. Use of the CrossBoss catheter (as described in Section 2.5.1) (Figure 4.17). The stent struts may act as a barrier preventing advancement of the CrossBoss catheter behind the restenosed stent, although occasionally the CrossBoss advancement may stop, requiring redirection with a guidewire (usually a polymer-jacketed guidewire, such as the Pilot 200).[20]
c. Retrograde crossing, as described in Chapter 6.

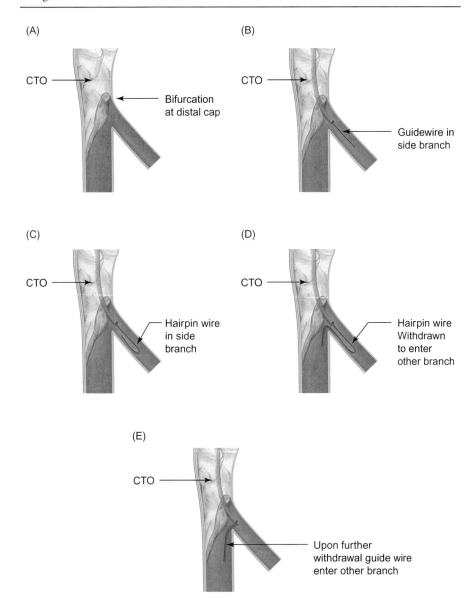

Figure 4.14 Technique for approaching CTOs after crossing into a side branch at the distal cap. A CTO with a bifurcation at the distal cap (A) is successfully crossed with a guidewire that enters the side branch (B). A hairpin guidewire is advanced into the side branch (C) and withdrawn, entering the main branch (D and E).

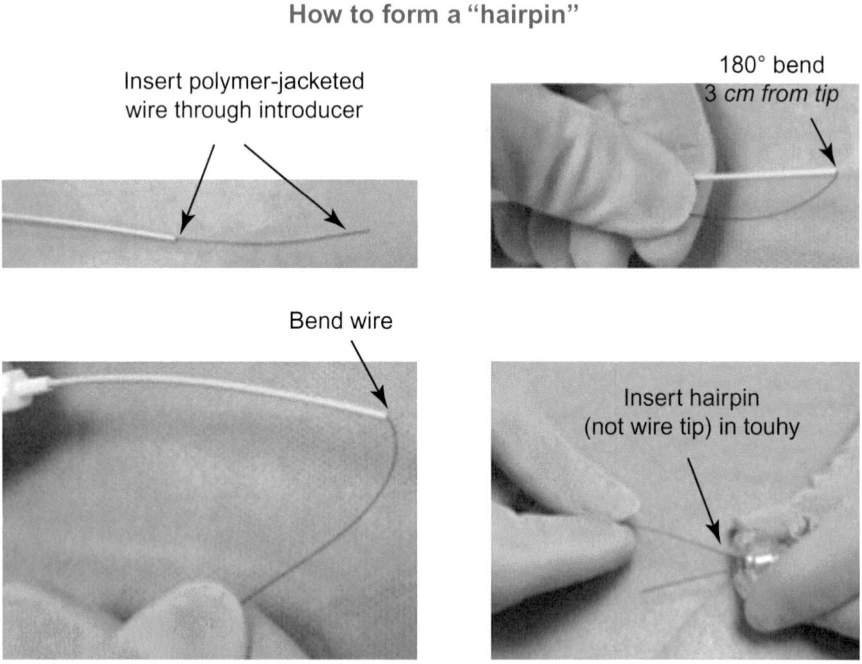

How to form a "hairpin"

Insert polymer-jacketed
wire through introducer

180° bend
3 cm from tip

Bend wire

Insert hairpin
(not wire tip) in touhy

Figure 4.15 Illustration of hairpin-wire creation.

4.1.6 Saphenous Vein Graft CTOs

Treatment of a saphenous vein graft (SVG) CTO is given a class III (level of evidence C) recommendation in the 2011 ACC/AHA PCI guidelines, due to high restenosis and repeat revascularization rates.[21] In patients with prior coronary bypass graft surgery treatment of a native coronary artery CTO is preferable to treatment of a SVG CTO supplying the same territory.[22] However, if native CTO PCI is not possible, PCI of the SVG CTO can provide a treatment option.[22–27]

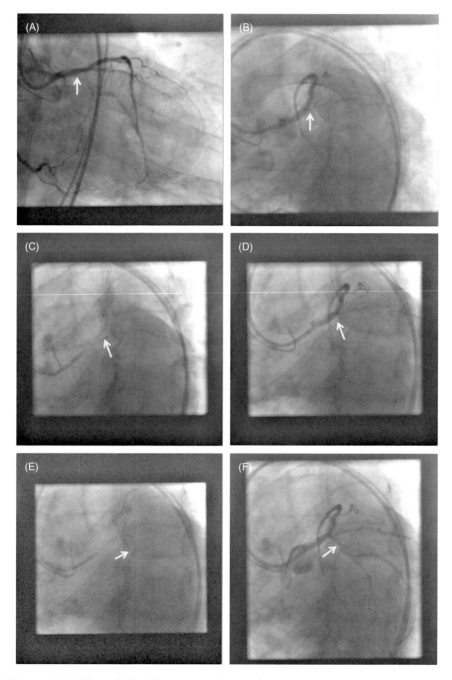

Figure 4.16 Use of the Venture catheter for treating an ostial circumflex occlusion. The case was complicated by stent loss. Bilateral

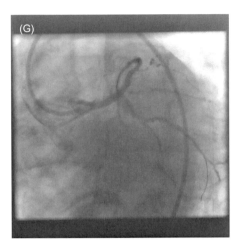

Figure 4.16 (Continued)

coronary angiography demonstrating an ostial chronic total occlusion of the circumflex (arrows, A and B). IVUS was performed to identify the ostium of the circumflex (arrow, C), followed by insertion of a Venture catheter (arrow, D), through which a Pilot 200 wire easily crossed the occlusion (arrow, E). After predilation antegrade flow in the circumflex was restored (arrow, F). In spite of multiple balloon predilations and use of a Guideliner catheter, a 2.5×23 mm³ stent could not be delivered and during attempts to retrieve it into the guide catheter it was dislodged from the balloon into the left main coronary artery. Attempts to retrieve the stent using a 4-mm Gooseneck snare were unsuccessful. During attempts to deliver a stent to the circumflex, the stent became dislodged and was crushed with another stent in the left main coronary artery followed by rewiring and balloon angioplasty of the circumflex with a satisfactory final angiographic result (G). This case highlights the value of the Venture catheter in highly angulated lesions, especially in ostial circumflex CTOs. The Venture catheter enabled rapid lesion crossing of a very challenging CTO in a tortuous and calcified vessel. In such vessels, stent delivery may also be very difficult and may be complicated by stent loss, as in this case. Aggressive lesion preparation may minimize the risk for stent loss.

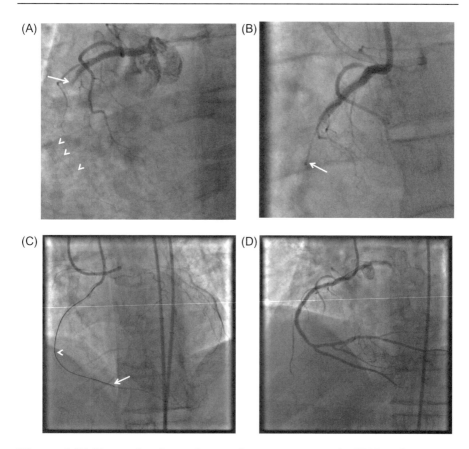

Figure 4.17 Example of treating an in-stent restenotic CTO using the CrossBoss catheter. Coronary angiography demonstrating a chronic total occlusion of the right coronary artery (arrow, A) due to in-stent restenosis (arrowheads, A). The CrossBoss catheter (arrow, B) was inserted into the lesion and advanced using the "fast spin" technique. The CrossBoss catheter could not be advanced through the stent (arrowhead, C), but a Confianza Pro 12 wire (arrow, C) crossed into the distal true lumen, as confirmed by contralateral injection. After stent implantation an excellent final result was achieved (D).
Source: Reproduced with permission from Ref. 20.

References

1. Grantham JA, Marso SP, Spertus J, House J, Holmes Jr. DR, Rutherford BD. Chronic total occlusion angioplasty in the United States. *JACC Cardiovasc Interv* 2009;**2**:479–86.
2. Morino Y, Kimura T, Hayashi Y, et al. In-hospital outcomes of contemporary percutaneous coronary intervention in patients with chronic total occlusion insights from the J-CTO Registry (Multicenter CTO Registry in Japan). *JACC Cardiovasc Interv* 2010;**3**:143–51.
3. Sianos G, Werner GS, Galassi AR, et al. Recanalisation of chronic total coronary occlusions: 2012 consensus document from the EuroCTO club. *EuroIntervention* 2012;**8**:139–45.
4. Brilakis ES, Grantham JA, Rinfret S, et al. A percutaneous treatment algorithm for crossing coronary chronic total occlusions. *JACC Cardiovasc Interv* 2012;**5**:367–79.
5. Rathore S, Matsuo H, Terashima M, et al. Procedural and in-hospital outcomes after percutaneous coronary intervention for chronic total occlusions of coronary arteries 2002 to 2008: impact of novel guidewire techniques. *JACC Cardiovasc Interv* 2009;**2**:489–97.
6. Mitsudo K, Yamashita T, Asakura Y, et al. Recanalization strategy for chronic total occlusions with tapered and stiff-tip guidewire. The results of CTO new techniQUE for STandard procedure (CONQUEST) trial. *J Invasive Cardiol* 2008;**20**:571–7.
7. Chiu CA. Recanalization of difficult bifurcation lesions using adjunctive double-lumen microcatheter support: two case reports. *J Invasive Cardiol* 2010;**22**:E99–103.
8. Saito S. Open Sesame Technique for chronic total occlusion. *Catheter Cardiovasc Interv* 2010;**75**:690–4.
9. Iturbe JM, Abdel-Karim AR, Raja VN, Rangan BV, Banerjee S, Brilakis ES. Use of the venture wire control catheter for the treatment of coronary artery chronic total occlusions. *Catheter Cardiovasc Interv* 2010;**76**:936–41.
10. Kawasaki T, Koga H, Serikawa T. New bifurcation guidewire technique: a reversed guidewire technique for extremely angulated bifurcation—a case report. *Catheter Cardiovasc Interv* 2008;**71**:73–6.
11. Suzuki G, Nozaki Y, Sakurai M. A novel guidewire approach for handling acute-angle bifurcations: reversed guidewire technique with adjunctive use of a double-lumen microcatheter. *J Invasive Cardiol* 2013;**25**:48–54.

12. Michael T, Banerjee S, Brilakis ES. Distal open sesame and hairpin wire techniques to facilitate a chronic total occlusion intervention. *J Invasive Cardiol* 2012;**24**:E57–9.
13. Abbas AE, Brewington SD, Dixon SR, Boura J, Grines CL, O'Neill WW. Success, safety, and mechanisms of failure of percutaneous coronary intervention for occlusive non-drug-eluting in-stent restenosis versus native artery total occlusion. *Am J Cardiol* 2005;**95**: 1462–6.
14. Yang YM, Mehran R, Dangas G, et al. Successful use of the frontrunner catheter in the treatment of in-stent coronary chronic total occlusions. *Catheter Cardiovasc Interv* 2004;**63**:462–8.
15. Ho PC. Treatment of in-stent chronic total occlusions with blunt microdissection. *J Invasive Cardiol* 2005;**17**:E37–9.
16. Lee NH, Cho YH, Seo HS. Successful recanalization of in-stent coronary chronic total occlusion by subintimal tracking. *J Invasive Cardiol* 2008;**20**:E129–32.
17. Werner GS, Moehlis H, Tischer K. Management of total restenotic occlusions. *EuroIntervention* 2009;**5**(Suppl. D):D79–83.
18. Brilakis ES, Lombardi WB, Banerjee S. Use of the Stingray guidewire and the Venture catheter for crossing flush coronary chronic total occlusions due to in-stent restenosis. *Catheter Cardiovasc Interv* 2010;**76**:391–4.
19. Abdel-karim AR, Lombardi WB, Banerjee S, Brilakis ES. Contemporary outcomes of percutaneous intervention in chronic total coronary occlusions due to in-stent restenosis. *Cardiovasc Revasc Med* 2011;**12**:170–6.
20. Papayannis A, Banerjee S, Brilakis ES. Use of the crossboss catheter in coronary chronic total occlusion due to in-stent restenosis. *Catheter Cardiovasc Interv* 2012;**80**:E30–6.
21. Levine GN, Bates ER, Blankenship JC, et al. ACCF/AHA/SCAI Guideline for Percutaneous Coronary Intervention. A report of the American College of Cardiology Foundation/American Heart Association Task Force on Practice Guidelines and the Society for Cardiovascular Angiography and Interventions. *J Am Coll Cardiol* 2011;**58**:e44–e122.
22. Brilakis ES, Banerjee S, Lombardi WL. Retrograde recanalization of native coronary artery chronic occlusions via acutely occluded vein grafts. *Catheter Cardiovasc Interv* 2010;**75**:109–13.
23. Sachdeva R, Uretsky BF. Retrograde recanalization of a chronic total occlusion of a saphenous vein graft. *Catheter Cardiovasc Interv* 2009;**74**:575–8.

24. Takano M, Yamamoto M, Mizuno K. A retrograde approach for the treatment of chronic total occlusion in a patient with acute coronary syndrome. *Int J Cardiol* 2007;**119**:e22−4.

25. Ho PC, Tsuchikane E. Improvement of regional ischemia after successful percutaneous intervention of bypassed native coronary chronic total occlusion: an application of the CART technique. *J Invasive Cardiol* 2008;**20**:305−8.

26. Brilakis ES, Grantham JA, Thompson CA, et al. The retrograde approach to coronary artery chronic total occlusions: a practical approach. *Catheter Cardiovasc Interv* 2012;**79**:3−19.

27. Garg N, Hakeem A, Gobal F, Uretsky BF. Outcomes of percutaneous coronary intervention of chronic total saphenous vein graft occlusions in the contemporary era. *Catheter Cardiovasc Interv* 2013. [Epub ahead of print]

5 Antegrade Dissection/Re-entry

Antegrade dissection/re-entry has emerged as a safe and efficient strategy for crossing long chronic total occlusions (CTOs), as outlined in the "hybrid" CTO crossing algorithm (Chapter 7). Antegrade dissection takes advantage of the distensibility of the subintimal space for traversing the occlusion rapidly and safely, concentrating subsequent efforts in crossing back into the distal true lumen (re-entry). In the past, distal true lumen re-entry was problematic because satisfactory tools and techniques were lacking, but dedicated equipment (Stingray balloon and guidewire, Boston Scientific) are currently available and have significantly facilitated re-entry.

Clarifying the Terminology (STAR, LAST, Mini-STAR, Contrast-Guided STAR)

The terminology utilized in dissection/re-entry CTO strategies can be confusing.[1] CTO crossing can occur either in the antegrade or in the retrograde direction. In either direction, crossing can be achieved either from true-to-true lumen or by first entering the subintimal space, followed by re-entry into the true lumen (dissection/re-entry strategies) (Figures 5.1 and 5.2).[1]

The term "subintimal" may increase this confusion, as there is typically no intimal layer within the atheroma of a totally occluded artery. Rather, "subintimal" in CTO PCI has evolved as a general term that refers to a tissue plane within or beyond the occlusion that may be (a) subintimal, (b) intraplaque, (c) intraadventitial, or (d) combinations thereof, where the location of a tissue plane is related to disease morphology and position along the length of the artery.

Manual of Coronary Chronic Total Occlusion Interventions. DOI: http://dx.doi.org/10.1016/B978-0-12-420129-3.00005-2

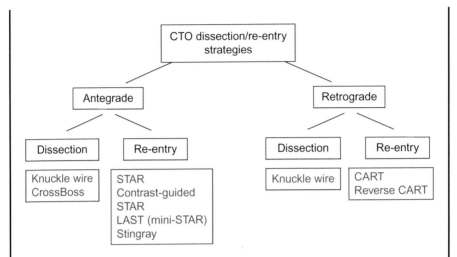

Figure 5.1 Classification of the CTO dissection/re-entry strategies.

Extensive dissection/re-entry (subintimal tracking and re-entry (STAR) technique), requires stenting of long coronary segments, often sacrifices side branches, and has been associated with poor long-term outcomes with high rates of in-stent restenosis.[2-4] The goal is always to achieve recanalization using limited dissection/ re-entry (with wire-based strategies or dedicated re-entry systems, such as the Stingray re-entry system) allowing targeted re-entry, side-branch preservation, and shorter stent lengths.

In the **antegrade** approach, dissection can be achieved by:

a. **Wire-based strategy, i.e., inadvertent wiring or knuckle wire**. A knuckle (prolapsed guidewire) is formed by pushing a polymer-jacketed guidewire (usually Fielder XT or Pilot 50 or 200) until it forms a "tight loop" at its tip (Figure 5.3). The knuckle is then advanced subintimally through the occlusion. Compared to trying to advance the tip of a wire, advancing a knuckle is much faster, safer (the tight loop minimizes the risk of vessel perforation), and less likely to enter side branches.

b. **Catheter-based strategy, using the CrossBoss catheter.**[5]

In the **antegrade** approach, re-entry can be achieved by:

1. **Wire-based strategy**
   a. Continuing to advance the knuckled guidewire until it spontaneously re-enters the true lumen (usually at a distal bifurcation).

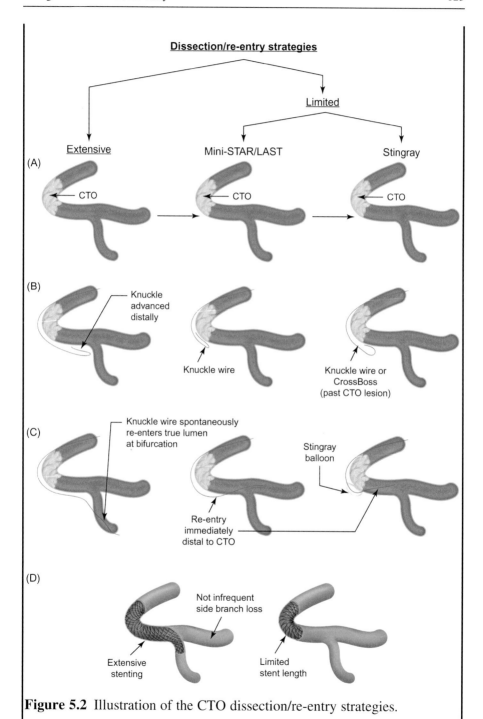

Figure 5.2 Illustration of the CTO dissection/re-entry strategies.

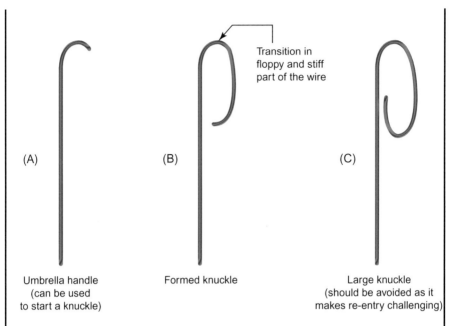

(A)   (B)   (C)

Umbrella handle   Formed knuckle   Large knuckle
(can be used   (should be avoided as it
to start a knuckle)   makes re-entry challenging)

Transition in
floppy and stiff
part of the wire

Figure 5.3 Illustration of knuckle wires. It is important to limit the diameter of the knuckle, as large knuckles enlarge the subintimal space and hinder re-entry.

This technique was introduced by Antonio Colombo and is called **STAR**.[2] A modification of the STAR technique called "contrast-guided STAR" by Mauro Carlino uses subintimal contrast injection through a microcatheter inserted into the proximal cap to create/visualize a dissection plane and facilitate guidewire advancement (Figure 5.4).[6] However, the STAR technique: (a) often results in side-branch loss, (b) is less predictably successful, (c) has high re-occlusion rates (likely due to long stent length and limited vessel outflow) and is rarely used as a definitive technique, but may be employed as a "last-ditch" effort, especially in the right coronary artery.[3]

b. Re-entering the true lumen as early as possible after the occlusion with a guidewire, which can be achieved by the "**mini-STAR**"[7] or the limited antegrade subintimal tracking (**LAST**)[8] technique (described in detail in Section 5.4.2). However, these techniques, tend to have lower success rates because of difficulty in reliably re-entering the true lumen, often due to extensive uncontrolled dissection with subintimal hematoma formation and true lumen compression.

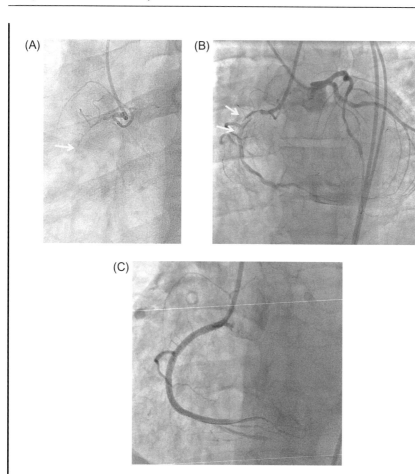

Figure 5.4 Contrast-guided STAR. CTO of the proximal right coronary artery (arrow, A), treated with injection of contrast via a microcatheter resulting in subintimal contrast entry (arrows, B) into the distal true lumen, with successful recanalization after stenting (C). *Source*: Reproduced with permission from Ref. 1.

2. Dedicated re-entry systems

> Using the **Stingray** (Boston Scientific) balloon and guidewire.[9–11]

In the **retrograde approach**, dissection is usually performed using a knuckle wire and re-entry is achieved using the techniques described in Chapter 6, Step 7.

Step 1 Decide that Antegrade Dissection/Re-Entry is the Next Step

Antegrade dissection/re-entry can be used:

a. As the initial crossing strategy (primary dissection/re-entry).
b. After failure of antegrade wire escalation (inadvertent subintimal wire crossing), or failure of the retrograde approach.

Good candidate lesions for primary dissection/re-entry strategy are those with:

a. Well-defined proximal cap.
b. ≥ 20 mm length.
c. Large caliber distal vessel.
d. No large branches within the CTO or, more importantly, at the distal cap.
e. Lack of good "interventional" collaterals.

Note

The optimal role and timing of antegrade dissection/re-entry in CTO PCI continues to be the subject of debate. "Hybrid" operators (Chapter 7) favor early application of antegrade dissection/re-entry to increase success rates and improve the efficiency of the procedure. Other operators argue that dissection/re-entry should only be used as a last resort after other crossing strategies fail, because the long-term patency of contemporary dissection/re-entry strategies remains unknown (similar to the retrograde dissection/re-entry techniques described in Section 6.7.2). Extensive dissection/re-entry techniques (such as STAR) have been associated with high restenosis and re-occlusion rates[3] and are infrequently used at present, except potentially as a final "bail-out" maneuver. To date there is limited data on the long-term outcomes with limited dissection/re-entry strategies.

Step 2 Getting to the CTO

Unless the CTO proximal cap is ostial or very proximal, it should be accessed with a workhorse guidewire advanced through a microcatheter, over-the-wire balloon, or CrossBoss catheter, as described in Chapter 4, Step 2.

Step 3 Subintimal Crossing: Knuckle Wire versus CrossBoss

Two techniques can be used for subintimal CTO crossing: (a) wire-based (knuckle wire technique) and (b) catheter-based (CrossBoss device).[9]
   The advantages of the CrossBoss catheter over a knuckle wire are that:

1. It creates a smaller more controlled subintimal dissection space, enabling a more predictable and controlled re-entry into the distal true lumen.
2. The relatively stiff CrossBoss catheter tends to advance along a longitudinal path parallel to the artery axis, whereas guidewires sometimes wrap around the artery circumference (in a "barber pole" fashion) hindering subsequent advancement of other devices and re-entry into the distal true lumen.

   In some cases both the CrossBoss catheter and a knuckle wire may be used ("knuckle-Boss" technique) to navigate beyond side branches or advance through calcific or tortuous anatomy.

5.1 Knuckle Wire

How to Knuckle a Wire

1. Use a polymer-jacketed wire (such as Fielder XT or Pilot 200—softer wires usually form smaller, tighter loops).
2. Can create "umbrella" bend using the introducer (this is not necessary, but is preferred, Figure 5.3A).
3. Push WITHOUT spinning (to minimize risk for wire fracture or entanglement).
4. Do not be afraid to push hard!
5. Loop usually forms at the junction of the radiopaque and the stiffer radiolucent parts of the wire (Figure 5.3B).

6. Try to keep the knuckle small—may need to withdraw into micro-catheter and re-advance if the knuckle size becomes too large (Figure 5.3C). Alternatively, the microcatheter can be advanced trying to keep the tip of the catheter as close as possible to the leading edge of the knuckle.
7. If a loop does not form, withdraw and re-advance.

What Can Go Wrong with the Knuckle

1. Can enter side branches.
2. Ensure knuckle is started within the subintimal space—do not start to knuckle if there are concerns that the wire is located outside the vessel "architecture," as this may cause a catastrophic perforation.
3. Knuckles (especially large ones) can cause extensive dissection and subintimal hematoma that can impair re-entry attempts. This can be prevented by crossing the distal CTO segment with the CrossBoss catheter ("**finish with the Boss**"), or by starting a knuckle in a more proximal location in the CTO target vessel.

5.2 CrossBoss

Step 1. The CrossBoss catheter is advanced into the proximal cap, and the workhorse guidewire is retracted within the catheter (Figure 5.5A).
Step 2. The CrossBoss catheter is rotated using a fast-spin technique and gentle forward pressure (Figure 5.5B). The catheter can be spun by hand in either direction, rotating as fast as possible. It is important to keep the CrossBoss torque device close to the hemostatic valve, as this prevents excessive advancement of the CrossBoss.
Step 3. After the CrossBoss advances forward, contralateral injection is performed to determine the distal CrossBoss position (Figure 5.5C).

What can go wrong?

a. CrossBoss fails to advance.
   i. Increase guide catheter support (e.g., by using a more supportive guide catheter, a side-branch anchor technique, or a guide catheter extension).

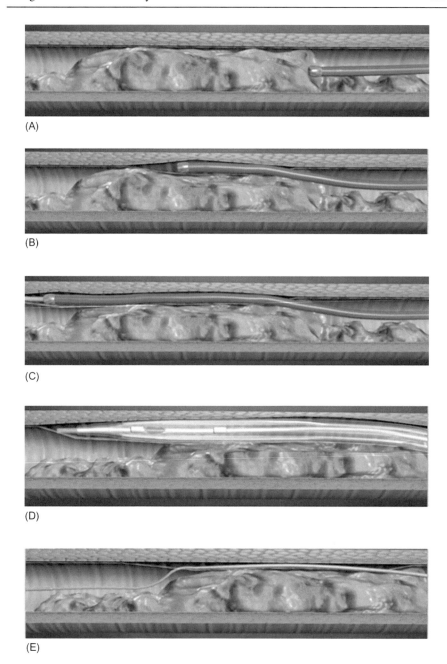

(A)

(B)

(C)

(D)

(E)

Figure 5.5 Illustration of use of the CrossBoss catheter and the Stingray guidewire.
Source: © 2013 Boston Scientific Corporation or its affiliates. All rights reserved. Used with permission of Boston Scientific Corporation.

ii. In patients with hard, calcified proximal cap, a stiff guidewire is used to puncture the proximal cap (should not be advanced >5−10 mm to prevent vessel perforation). This wire should be immediately withdrawn and the CrossBoss advanced by itself, using the fast-spin technique. Alternatively, a polymer-jacketed wire could be used to create a knuckle and subsequently advanced, followed by CrossBoss crossing of the final CTO segment.

b. CrossBoss enters side branch.

i. It is very important to detect this course of the CrossBoss catheter using imaging in various projections with contralateral injection, as continued CrossBoss advancement through a side branch can lead to perforation.

ii. The CrossBoss catheter is retracted and redirected using a stiff guidewire (such as Confianza Pro 12) or a knuckle wire, which is less likely to enter the side branches.

iii. The CrossBoss catheter may also be advanced once it reaches the distal portion of the knuckle ("knuckle-Boss" technique).

CrossBoss: Tips and Tricks

1. The CrossBoss catheter may cross into the distal true lumen in approximately one-third of cases (Figure 5.6).

2. Rapid rotation in either or both directions is key while advancing the CrossBoss catheter, as it reduces friction between catheter and tissue. Only gentle forward pressure should be applied.

3. Excellent guide support is critical for enhancing the CrossBoss catheter crossing success.

4. After subintimal crossing with the CrossBoss it is useful to disconnect the contrast-containing syringe from the antegrade guide catheter manifold (or cover the manifold) to minimize the risk of hydraulic dissection. Inadvertent contrast injection could enlarge the subintimal space and hinder re-entry attempts (Figure 5.7).

5. The torque device is usually attached 2−3 cm (three finger widths) proximal to the Y-connector, to limit potentially excessive forward movement of the CrossBoss catheter (so-called "CrossBoss jump"). As the CrossBoss catheter engages and penetrates tissue, at times the device stores torsional energy and has the propensity to jump during advancement and navigation. There are three possible outcomes after a CrossBoss jump: (1) CTO yield and advancement into

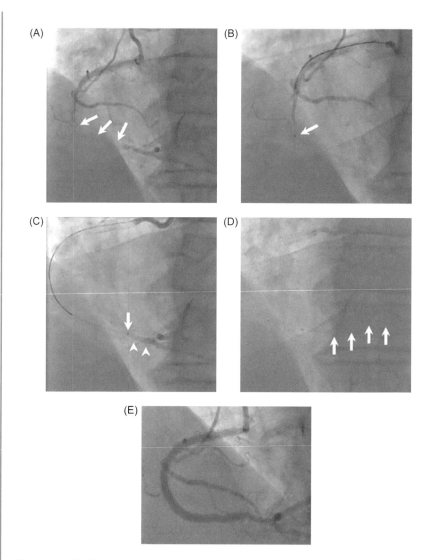

Figure 5.6 Example of true-to-true lumen crossing using the CrossBoss catheter. Previously failed CTO of a right coronary artery (arrows, A) with CrossBoss catheter tip (arrows, B and C) crossing to the distal true lumen (arrowheads, C), facilitating distal wire placement (arrows, D), predilation, and an excellent final result (E).

Source: Reproduced with permission from Ref. 5.

(A)

(B)

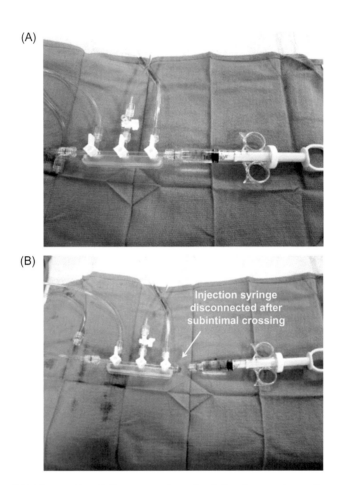

Injection syringe
disconnected after
subintimal crossing

Figure 5.7 Example of disconnecting the injection syringe from the manifold (B) after antegrade subintimal crossing to prevent inadvertent contrast injection that could enlarge the subintimal space.

the distal true lumen, (2) advancement into a side branch, or (3) exit from the vessel. This is why forward movement is best limited by having the torque device attached close to the Y-connector, thus limiting the length of catheter that may be introduced into the body.

6. The CrossBoss should be removed over a stiff, straight, non-lubricious guide wire, such as a Miracle 12, using the trapping technique to prevent wire movement and maintain distal position without enlarging the dissection.

Step 4 Re-entry into Distal True Lumen

After subintimal CTO crossing has been achieved, re-entry into the distal true lumen can be achieved using: (a) dedicated re-entry systems, such as the Stingray system, or (b) guidewire-based techniques.

5.3   Stingray-Based Re-entry

Step 1 Preparation of the Stingray Balloon

- **Stingray preparation steps** (Figure 5.8):

    1. Attach a new, completely dry, three-way stopcock to the end of the Stingray balloon port (Figure 5.8A).
    2. Using a new, completely dry 20 cc luer-lock syringe, aspirate negative 2—3 times (Figure 5.8B) and turn stopcock (Figure 5.8C), to retain vacuum in the Stingray balloon.
    3. Remove the 20-cc syringe, replacing it with a 3-cc luer-lock syringe that contains 100% contrast (Figure 5.8D).
    4. Flush contrast through three-way stopcock, ensuring that there are no air bubbles (Figure 5.8E).
    5. Open stopcock to syringe—the plunger will advance by 2—3 mm (Figure 5.8F is before opening stopcock; Figure 5.8G is after opening stopcock).
    6. The Stingray balloon is now ready for use (Figure 5.8H).

Step 2 Delivery of the Stingray Balloon to the Re-entry Zone (Figure 5.5D)

Stingray balloon delivery is usually easy if the CrossBoss or a knuckle wire was used to create the dissection. If subintimal wire position was achieved during antegrade wire escalation, then predilation of the subintimal space at the CTO segment may need to be performed to facilitate delivery of the Stingray balloon to the re-entry segment. Occasionally, while trying to deliver the Stingray balloon to the re-entry zone, the guidewire may enter the distal true lumen. Alternatively, strategies to increase guide catheter support (guide catheter extension or side-branch anchor) can be used. Stingray balloon delivery can also be facilitated by using a supportive guidewire for delivery, such as a 300-cm-long Miracle 12 guidewire. It is

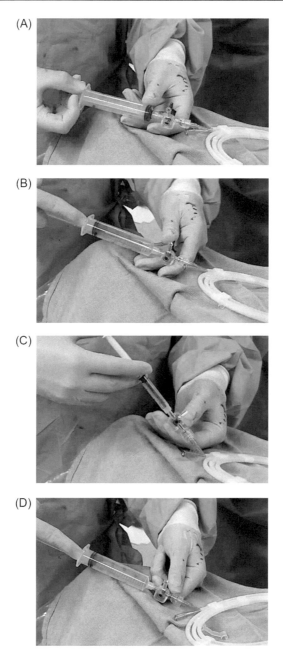

Figure 5.8 Illustration of the Stingray balloon preparation.

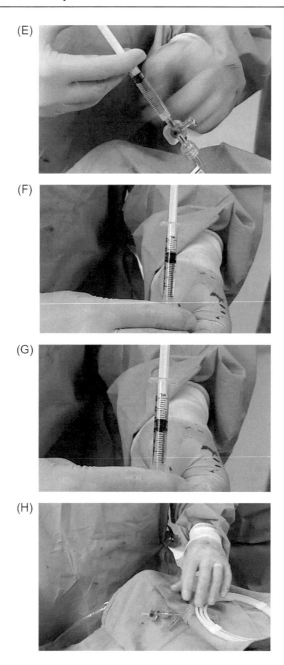

Figure 5.8 (Continued)

recommended that the wire-trapping technique be used to avoid inadvertent movement of the exchange wire. Of note, trapping cannot be performed with the Stingray balloon through 7 Fr guide catheters; it can only be performed with 8 Fr guide catheters).

Step 3 Re-entry into the Distal True Lumen

After the Stingray balloon is delivered to the re-entry zone, it is inflated at 2—4 atm. Orthogonal angiographic projections are then obtained to select the optimal view for re-entry (Figure 5.9). The ideal view is the one in which the Stingray balloon is seen as one line located at the side of the vessel lumen (Figure 5.9B). The side view is necessary to determine in which direction the wire leaves the Stingray balloon, so as to direct it toward the vessel lumen.

To re-enter the distal true lumen the Stingray guidewire is advanced through the Stingray balloon side ports under fluoroscopic guidance. The Stingray balloon has three exit ports: two 180° apart for vessel re-entry and an end hole. The proximal exit port is proximal to the two markers, and the other exit port is between the two markers. If the

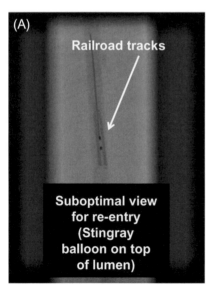 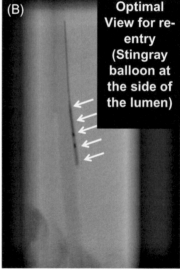

Figure 5.9 Selection of the optimal view to facilitate re-entry using the Stingray balloon.

wire enters the exit port that faces away from the true lumen, it is withdrawn and redirected into the other exit port facing the true lumen.

Once the wire is in the correct port, it is advanced without rotation so as to puncture back into the true lumen. This often creates a "pop" sensation. Contralateral injection is now helpful to determine whether true lumen re-entry has been achieved. If this is the case and the distal vessel is not severely diseased and the lumen is large, the Stingray guidewire can be rotated 180° and advanced further down into the vessel (Figure 5.5E). This is also called the "**stick-and-drive**" method.

An example of successful Stingray-based re-entry is demonstrated in Figure 5.10.

Step 4 Exchange for a Workhorse Wire

The Stingray wire has a stiff, highly penetrating distal tip, hence it should be replaced after successful CTO crossing to minimize the risk for distal vessel injury during balloon angioplasty and stenting. This is accomplished by advancing a balloon or microcatheter over the Stingray wire after the Stingray balloon has been removed (preferably using the trapping technique if 8 Fr guide catheters are used), withdrawal of the Stingray wire, and insertion of a workhorse guidewire.

What can go wrong?

1. **Unable to advance Stingray balloon to the re-entry zone**
   If the Stingray cannot be delivered to the re-entry zone, the following steps could be performed:
   a. Balloon angioplasty with a small (1.2–1.5 mm) balloon.
   b. Use of techniques to enhance guide catheter support, such as anchoring techniques or guide catheter extensions.
2. **Poor visualization of the Stingray balloon and the distal true lumen**
   Potential solutions:
   a. Meticulous preparation of the Stingray balloon.
   b. Orthogonal views to identify optimal re-entry projection: the goal is to achieve a "sideways" projection (Figure 5.9B) and avoid a "railroad projection" (Figure 5.9A).
   c. Magnified views (which is discouraged during the other parts of the CTO PCI procedure to reduce radiation dose).

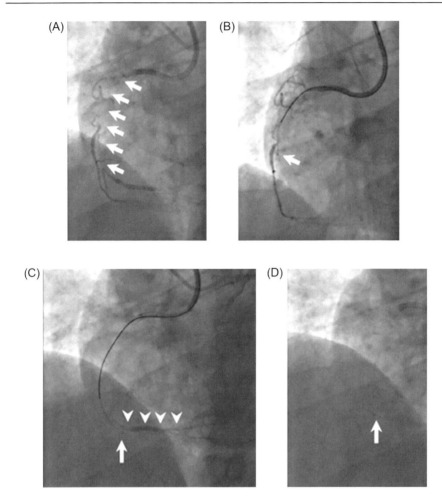

Figure 5.10 Successful re-entry into the distal true lumen using the Stingray balloon and wire. CTO of a right coronary artery (arrows, A) with CrossBoss catheter tip (arrows, B and C) crossing into the false lumen (true lumen, arrowheads, E) followed by Stingray catheter placement (arrow, D), Stingray guidewire re-entry (arrow, E) through the Stingray catheter into the distal true lumen (arrows, F), predilation, and final result (G).
Source: Reproduced with permission from Ref. 5.

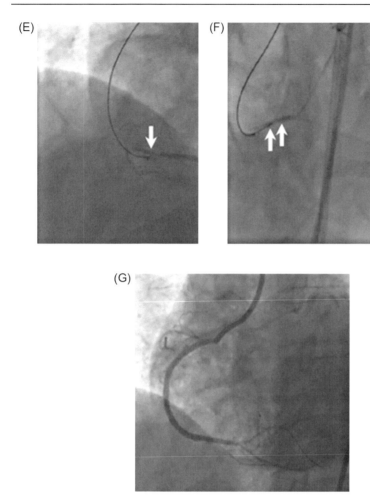

Figure 5.10 (Continued)

3. Unable to enter diffusely diseased distal vessel

Re-entry from the subintimal space into the distal true lumen can be difficult in patients with small, diffusely diseased distal vessels, because the re-entry lumen is small and the Stingray wire may go "through and through" the true lumen into the opposite vessel wall (Figure 5.11A).

Solutions:

a. Change re-entry site by moving the Stingray balloon to a healthier, straighter, and larger vessel segment (the horizontal part of the distal right coronary artery is usually preferable for re-entry).

(A)

(B)

(C)

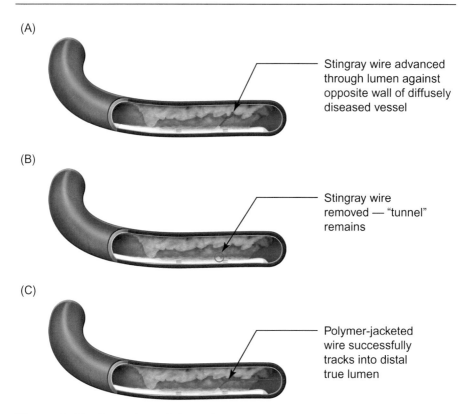

Stingray wire advanced through lumen against opposite wall of diffusely diseased vessel

Stingray wire removed — "tunnel" remains

Polymer-jacketed wire successfully tracks into distal true lumen

Figure 5.11 Illustration of the "stick-and-swap" technique.

b. Use the **"Stick-and-Swap"** technique (Figure 5.11): an initial puncture is performed using the Stingray wire to create a connection with the distal true lumen (A). The Stingray wire is removed (B), and a Pilot 200 (or similar polymer-jacketed) guidewire is advanced through the same side port into the "tunnel" created by the Stingray wire. The (A) polymer-jacketed guidewire is more likely to track into the distal vessel lumen successfully completing the re-entry maneuver (C).

4. **Compression of distal true lumen by hematoma**
   Prevention of subintimal hematoma is key to successful re-entry. Use of the CrossBoss catheter (rather than a knuckle wire) for dissection (especially in the distal segment of the occlusion) can reduce the risk compared to a knuckle wire. If a hematoma develops, then aspiration of the hematoma can be attempted, either through the Stingray balloon itself, or ideally through another microcatheter or over-the-wire balloon advanced next to

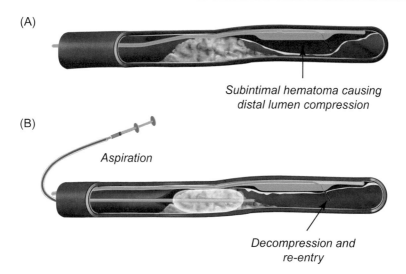

(A)

Subintimal hematoma causing
distal lumen compression

(B)

Aspiration

Decompression and
re-entry

Figure 5.12 Illustration of the STRAW technique. (A) demonstrates subintimal hematoma that compressed the distal true lumen, hindering re-entry attempts with the Stingray balloon and guidewire. (B) shows insertion of a second over-the-wire balloon advanced into the subintimal space, through which aspiration is performed decompressing the hematoma and allowing re-expansion of the distal true lumen facilitating re-entry.

the Stingray balloon. This is called the **STRAW** (Subintimal Transcatheter Withdrawal) technique (Figures 5.12 and 5.13). This technique can only be performed when using an 8-Fr guide catheter. A modified STRAW technique can be performed by advancing a guide extension, such as a Guideliner catheter (Vascular Solutions), into the vessel and aspirating at the manifold. The STRAW technique is most effective if the proximal vessel is occluded (e.g., with a balloon) to prevent continuing expansion from proximal blood flow.

5. **Distal vessel calcification**

   Re-entry can be challenging in densely calcified vessels. Potential solutions:

   a. Use a different, stiff, tapered, highly penetrating guidewire, such as a Confianza Pro 12 guidewire (Asahi Intecc), to make a puncture through the calcified vessel wall.

   b. Attempt re-entry into a more distal location (by advancing the Stingray balloon—this is often called the "**bobsled**" technique).

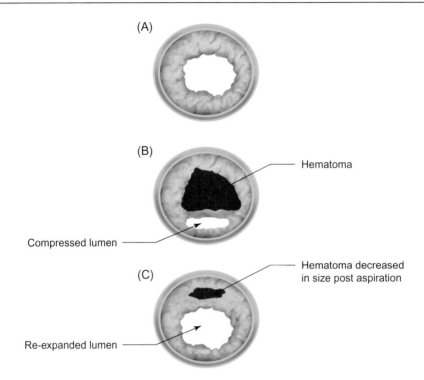

(A)

(B)

Hematoma

Compressed lumen

Hematoma decreased
in size post aspiration

(C)

Re-expanded lumen

**Figure 5.13 Cross-sections of the vessel illustrating the STRAW
technique.** (A) demonstrates the CTO vessel distal to the occlusion. (B)
demonstrates the effect of hematoma formation in the subintimal space with
compression of the distal true lumen. (C) illustrates re-expansion of the
distal true lumen after aspiration of the hematoma, which facilitates
guidewire re-entry.

6. Occlusion of side branch at distal cap

Problem: Re-entry into one of the branches at the distal CTO cap
can result in occlusion of the other branch.
Solutions:
a. Re-enter proximal to the bifurcation, which is usually accomplished
using a stiff, penetrating guidewire.
b. Enter one vessel and refenestrate the other using a stiff guidewire in order to be more precise, or change to a mini-STAR
technique. Sometimes, one may need to use the retrograde
approach to restore patency of the other vessel (Figure 5.14).

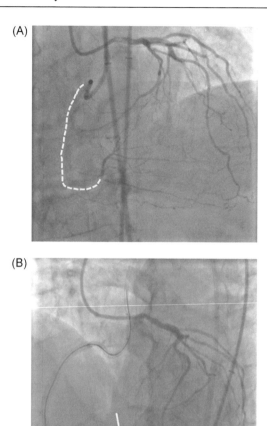

Figure 5.14 Example of using the retrograde approach for preserving both branches of a bifurcation at the distal CTO cap. PCI of a long (dotted line, A) right coronary artery CTO was attempted. Antegrade crossing into the right posterolateral vessel (PLV, arrow, B) was achieved using a CrossBoss catheter and a Pilot 200 and Confianza Pro 12 guidewire. Antegrade flow was restored into the PLV after balloon predilation, but several attempts to antegradely wire the right posterior descending artery (PDA) failed. Retrograde crossing into the right PDA via a septal collateral was then performed (C).

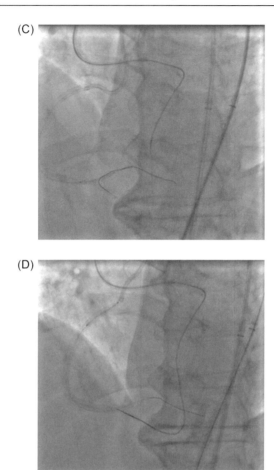

Figure 5.14 (Continued.)

◄ After stenting into the PLV antegradely, retrograde crossing into the distal
RCA was performed with a Confianza Pro 12 guidewire (D and E),
followed by wire externalization and PDA stenting (F) using a mini-crush
technique. An excellent final angiographic result was achieved with
preservation of flow into both PDA and PLV (arrows, G).

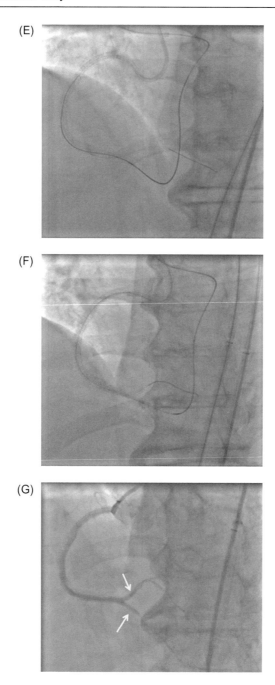

Figure 5.14 (Continued.)

5.4 Wire-Based Re-entry

Although use of the Stingray balloon and guidewire is the preferred, more controlled, re-entry technique, if it is not available or
if it fails to achieve re-entry, wire-based re-entry techniques can
be used.

5.4.1 STAR

Step 1: The re-entry guidewire (usually polymer-jacketed, such as Pilot
50 or 200 or Fielder XT or FC) is inserted within the lesion and a loop is
formed at the distal tip.

Step 2: The knuckled guidewire is advanced until it spontaneously re-enters
the true lumen (usually at a distal bifurcation).[7] This may be easier to
accomplish than more limited wire re-entry or Stingray re-entry techniques.

What can go wrong

a. Extensive shearing and occlusion of side branches, resulting in limited
   outflow. The STAR technique should NOT be used in the left anterior
   descending artery, as it will lead to significant loss of the septal and
   diagonal branches (and may also preclude future coronary bypass graft
   surgery due to extensive stent implantation).
b. Inability to re-enter the distal true lumen. If this occurs then use of the
   Stingray system may facilitate re-entry, although re-entry will likely continue to be challenging because of the extensive dissection caused by the
   STAR technique.
c. High restenosis and re-occlusion rates (likely due to the long stent length
   and limited outflow, although studies are limited by presenting data with
   both drug-eluting and bare-metal stents and considering TIMI 2 flow
   post PCI as successful procedure):
   • 52% need for target vessel revascularization in the original Colombo
     series.[2]
   • 54% restenosis with contrast-guided STAR.[4]
   • 57% re-occlusion rate in an Italian registry.[3]

In summary, the STAR technique should be used only as a last
resort option in CTO PCI due to loss of side branches and high restenosis rates.

5.4.2 LAST or Mini-STAR (Figures 5.15−5.18)

Step 1. The antegrade microcatheter is advanced into the CTO lesion.

Step 2. The re-entry guidewire is selected. In "mini-STAR,"[7] the Fielder FC or XT wire is used. In LAST re-entry, a Pilot 200 or a Confianza Pro 12 guidewire is used.

Step 3. The re-entry guidewire is shaped to facilitate re-entry, as follows (Figure 5.15):

Mini-STAR: A 40−50° curve is created 1−2 mm proximal to the tip and a second 15−20° curve is created 3−5 mm proximal to the tip.

LAST: A 90° curve is created 2−3 mm proximal to the tip.

Step 4. The re-entry wire is manipulated until re-entry is achieved into the distal true lumen. This can be occasionally facilitated by use of the Venture wire control catheter[12] or the Twin-Pass dual lumen catheter.

What can go wrong

a. Failure to re-enter—other techniques (such as the Stingray system and retrograde crossing) can be used in these cases.

b. Distal true lumen compression by subintimal hematoma. Use of the STRAW technique (Figures 5.12 and 5.13) can be used to decompress the hematoma.

c. Wire perforation: Wire perforation alone will only rarely cause tamponade, but it is important to detect it early to prevent advancement of equipment, such as balloons and microcathethers, which will enlarge the exit point and may cause a catastrophic perforation.

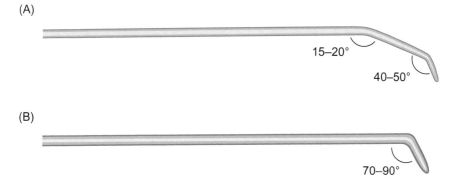

(A)

15–20°

40–50°

(B)

70–90°

Figure 5.15 Illustration of the wire bends used for the mini-STAR (A) and the LAST (B) techniques.

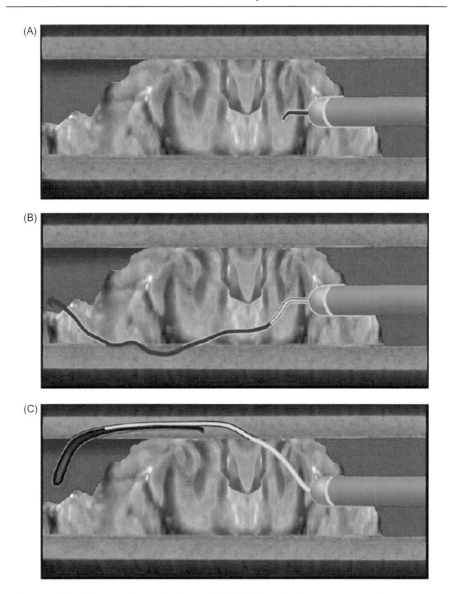

Figure 5.16 Illustration of the mini-STAR technique. (A): The microcatheter is advanced into the CTO body and the initial wire is exchanged with a Fielder FC wire (Asahi Intec). The Fielder FC wire is pushed against the CTO achieving recanalization of the occluded vessel by navigation in an intra- or extravascular microchannel (B) or via small subintimal tracking with an auto J-shape configuration (C).

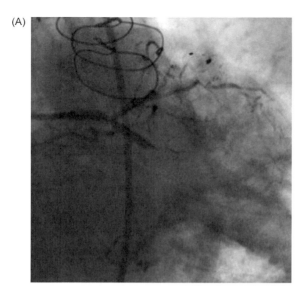

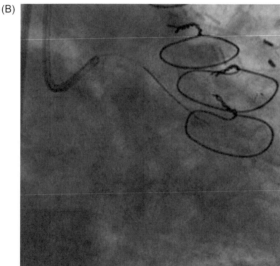

Figure 5.17 Example of the mini-STAR technique. (A): Left circumflex (LCX) CTO with faint ipsilateral collateral circulation that was approached with a Confianza guidewire (Asahi Intec) through a Finecross microcatheter (Terumo). (B): The stiff guidewire could not cross and was exchanged for a Fielder FC guidewire (Asahi Intecc). (C): The Fielder FC wire was gently advanced toward the occlusion, creating a large loop close to its tip. (D): The guidewire was advanced further, achieving subintimal crossing of the occlusion. (E): Re-entry of the Fielder FC guidewire into the distal true lumen after the distal cap. (F): Final result after four-drug-eluting stent implantation, with reconstruction of the circumflex/obtuse marginal bifurcation using a mini-crush technique.
Source: Courtesy of Dr. Alfredo Galassi.

(C)

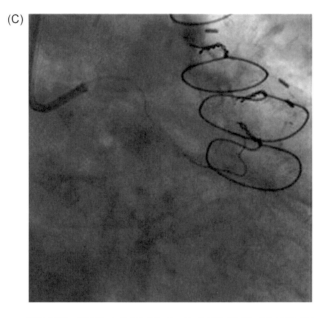

(D)

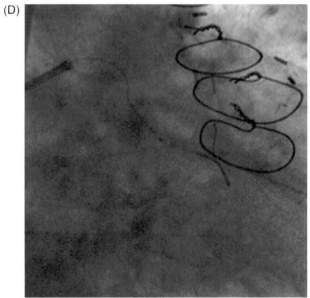

Figure 5.17 (Continued.)

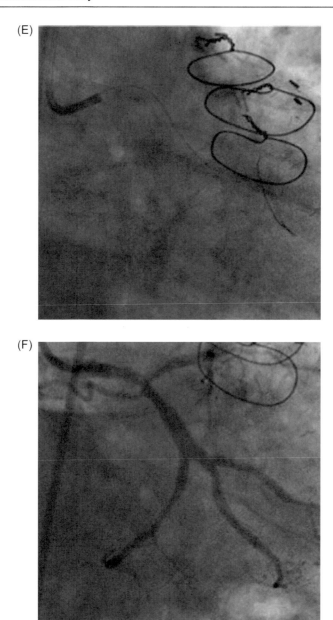

Figure 5.17 (Continued.)

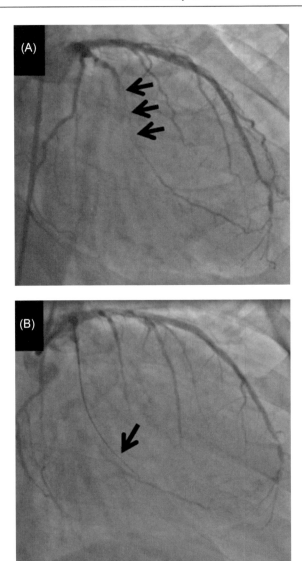

Figure 5.18 Example of the LAST technique. CTO of the ramus
intermedius branch (arrows, A). Crossing attempts with a Confianza Pro 12
wire (Abbott Vascular) failed (arrow, B). A Fielder XT wire (Asahi Intecc)
remained intraluminal but could not cross the occlusion (arrow, C). The
Fielder XT wire was advanced until a knuckle formed at its tip (arrow, D—
notice the small size of the knuckle) that crossed the CTO into the
subintimal space. A Confianza Pro 12 guidewire with a 90° distal bend was
used to re-enter into the distal true lumen (LAST technique—arrow, E),
with an excellent final angiographic result post-stenting (F).
Source: Reproduced with permission from Ref. 1.

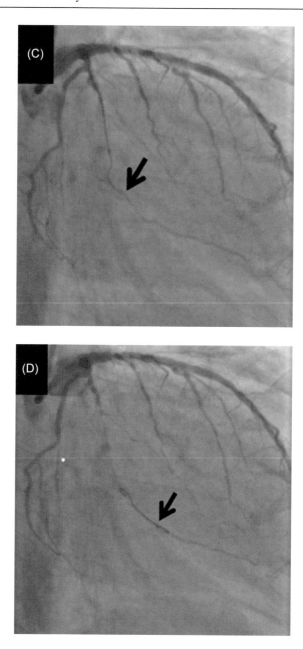

Figure 5.18 (Continued.)

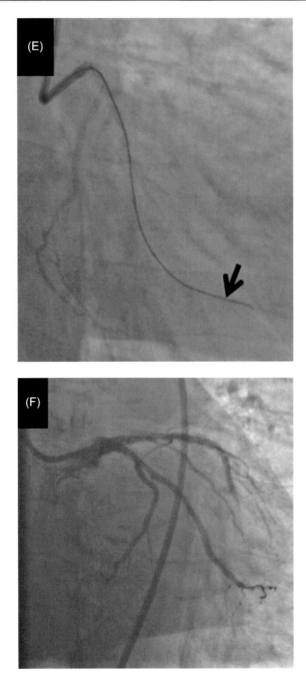

Figure 5.18 (Continued.)

References

1. Michael TT, Papayannis AC, Banerjee S, Brilakis ES. Subintimal dissection/reentry strategies in coronary chronic total occlusion interventions. *Circ Cardiovasc Interv* 2012;**5**:729−38.
2. Colombo A, Mikhail GW, Michev I, et al. Treating chronic total occlusions using subintimal tracking and reentry: the STAR technique. *Catheter Cardiovasc Interv* 2005;**64**:407−11.
3. Valenti R, Vergara R, Migliorini A, et al. Predictors of reocclusion after successful drug-eluting stent-supported percutaneous coronary intervention of chronic total occlusion. *J Am Coll Cardiol* 2013;**61**: 545−50.
4. Godino C, Latib A, Economou FI, et al. Coronary chronic total occlusions: mid-term comparison of clinical outcome following the use of the guided-STAR technique and conventional anterograde approaches. *Catheter Cardiovasc Interv* 2012;**79**:20−7.
5. Whitlow PL, Burke MN, Lombardi WL, et al. Use of a novel crossing and re-entry system in coronary chronic total occlusions that have failed standard crossing techniques: results of the FAST-CTOs (Facilitated Antegrade Steering Technique in Chronic Total Occlusions) trial. *JACC Cardiovasc Interv* 2012;**5**:393−401.
6. Carlino M, Godino C, Latib A, Moses JW, Colombo A. Subintimal tracking and re-entry technique with contrast guidance: a safer approach. *Catheter Cardiovasc Interv* 2008;**72**:790−6.
7. Galassi AR, Tomasello SD, Costanzo L, et al. Mini-STAR as bail-out strategy for percutaneous coronary intervention of chronic total occlusion. *Catheter Cardiovasc Interv* 2012;**79**:30−40.
8. Lombardi WL. Retrograde PCI: what will they think of next? *J Invasive Cardiol* 2009;**21**:543.
9. Werner GS. The BridgePoint devices to facilitate recanalization of chronic total coronary occlusions through controlled subintimal reentry. *Expert Rev Med Devices* 2011;**8**:23−9.
10. Brilakis ES, Lombardi WB, Banerjee S. Use of the Stingray guidewire and the Venture catheter for crossing flush coronary chronic total occlusions due to in-stent restenosis. *Catheter Cardiovasc Interv* 2010;**76**:391−4.
11. Brilakis ES, Badhey N, Banerjee S. "Bilateral knuckle" technique and Stingray re-entry system for retrograde chronic total occlusion intervention. *J Invasive Cardiol* 2011;**23**:E37−9.
12. Badhey N, Lombardi WL, Thompson CA, Brilakis ES, Banerjee S. Use of the venture wire control catheter for subintimal coronary dissection and reentry in chronic total occlusions. *J Invasive Cardiol* 2010;**22**: 445−8.

6 The Retrograde Approach

6.1 Historical Perspective

The retrograde technique differs from the standard antegrade approach in that the occlusion is approached from the distal vessel advancing a wire against the original direction of blood flow, i.e., retrograde.[1,2] The guidewire is advanced into the artery distal to the occlusion through either a bypass graft or a collateral channel. This approach differs from the antegrade approach, in which all equipment is inserted only proximal to the occlusion and travels in the same direction as the original arterial flow, i.e., antegrade.

The retrograde chronic total occlusion (CTO) percutaneous coronary intervention (PCI) technique was first described in 1990 by Kahn and Hartzler, who performed balloon angioplasty of a left anterior descending artery (LAD) CTO via a saphenous vein graft (SVG).[3] In 1996, Silvestri et al. reported retrograde stenting of the left main artery via a SVG.[4] In 2006, Surmely et al. reported for the first time retrograde crossing via septal collaterals,[5] starting the modern era of the retrograde techniques through septal[5–10] and epicardial[11] collaterals and arterial bypass grafts.[10] The introduction of specialized equipment and further refinements of the technique started in Japan[12,13] with rapid adoption both in Europe[14–16] and in the United States.[17,18]

6.2 Advantages of the Retrograde Approach

Crossing in the retrograde direction can sometimes be easier than antegrade crossing because the distal cap:

a. Is easier to enter than the proximal cap, as it is more frequently tapered.

Manual of Coronary Chronic Total Occlusion Interventions. DOI: http://dx.doi.org/10.1016/B978-0-12-420129-3.00006-4

b. Is often softer than the proximal cap, likely because of exposure to lower filling pressure.

c. Is less frequently anatomically ambiguous.

Moreover, the antegrade approach may not be feasible in some CTOs, e.g., ostial and stumpless CTOs, CTOs with ambiguous proximal cap, or long and tortuous CTOs.

6.3 Special Equipment

In addition to the standard equipment needed for the antegrade approach, the retrograde approach requires specialized equipment, i.e., short guides, specialized microcatheters (150-cm-long Corsair), long guidewires for externalization, such as the Viper, R350, and RG3 (the RG3 is not currently available in the United States) wires, and guidewires for crossing the collateral vessels, as described in Chapter 2.

a. Short guide catheters

The standard guide catheter length is 100 cm (shaft length, although the length from the hub to the guide tip is approximately 106 cm).[1] If standard guide catheters are used for the retrograde approach, equipment may not be long enough to reach the lesion retrogradely and wires advanced retrogradely may be too short to be externalized. Utilizing a shorter guide catheter extends the reach of balloons, wires, and microcatheters advanced retrogradely, as most of the catheter outside the body has been removed by the shorter guide length. Short guide catheters (80, 85, or 90 cm) are commercially available, but if they are not locally available, any guide can be shortened using a interposition segment of a sheath, as described in Section 2.2.2 and Figure 2.2.[19]

b. Microcatheters

The Corsair channel dilator is important for the retrograde approach, as it facilitates collateral crossing and provides collateral dilation at the same time, obviating the need for separate balloon dilation of septal collaterals (epicardial collaterals can be crossed with the Corsair catheter **but should never be dilated with a balloon**). The Corsair catheter construction is described in detail in Section 2.3.2). If a Corsair catheter is not available, other microcatheters, such as the 150-cm-long Finecross can also be used, as described in Section 2.3.3.

c. Long guidewires

Long guidewires are important for externalization, as standard length guidewires are too short. The technical characteristics of the externalization guidewires are described in detail in Section 2.4.5.

d. Collateral crossing guidewires

Preferred wires for septal crossing have traditionally been soft, polymer-jacketed wires such as the Fielder FC. Lately, composite core hydrophilic wires, such as the Sion wire, have shown even better performance in channel tracking, especially in small and very tortuous collaterals. The tip bend should be very short (1 mm) and quite shallow (20−30°) to allow for tracking very small, tortuous collaterals.

6.4 Step-by-Step Description of the Procedure

Step 1 Decide that Retrograde Is the Next Step

Goal: Decide when the retrograde approach should be used.

How?

A. Appropriate collaterals exist.

And

B. There is local experience and expertise in the retrograde technique.

And

C1. The antegrade approach fails.

Or

C2. As the initial crossing strategy (primary retrograde) in the following cases:

1. Ambiguous proximal cap or "stumpless" occlusions.
2. Ostial occlusions.[20,21]
3. Long occlusions.
4. Severe proximal tortuosity or calcification.
5. Small or poorly visualized distal vessel.
6. CTO vessels that are difficult to engage, such as anomalous coronary arteries.[20,22]
7. Occlusion involving a distal major bifurcation.
8. Patients with impaired renal function, as the retrograde approach may require less contrast than the antegrade approach.

Step 2 Selecting the Collateral

Goal: Select the collateral(s) that will be used for the retrograde approach.

How?

The usual preference order for selecting a retrograde collateral channel is bypass graft, septal, and then epicardial. The advantages and disadvantages of each collateral channel are shown in Figure 6.1.[1] The classification and optimal angiographic views for evaluating collateral vessels are discussed in detail in Section 3.3.2.

Bypass grafts are large and easy to wire (Figure 6.2). Prior coronary bypass graft surgery causes scarring of the pericardium and reduces (but does not eliminate[23]) the likelihood of free pericardial effusion and tamponade in case of perforation during CTO PCI. Even acutely occluded SVGs can serve as conduits to the distal arterial segment of chronically occluded native coronary arteries.[24] There is currently controversy as to whether degenerated SVGs used as retrograde conduit for CTO PCI should be coiled after successful completion of CTO PCI. Coiling could stop competitive flow through the native stented segment and possibly decrease the risk of subsequent stent occlusion or thrombosis.

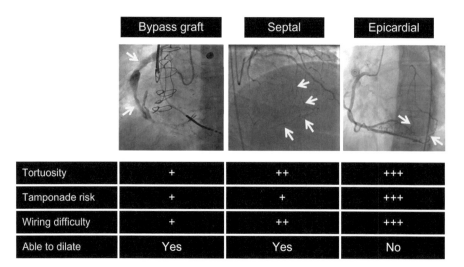

	Bypass graft	Septal	Epicardial
Tortuosity	+	++	+++
Tamponade risk	+	+	+++
Wiring difficulty	+	++	+++
Able to dilate	Yes	Yes	No

Figure 6.1 Comparison of advantages and disadvantages of various collateral vessels that can be used for retrograde CTO interventions. *Source*: Modified with permission from Ref. 1.

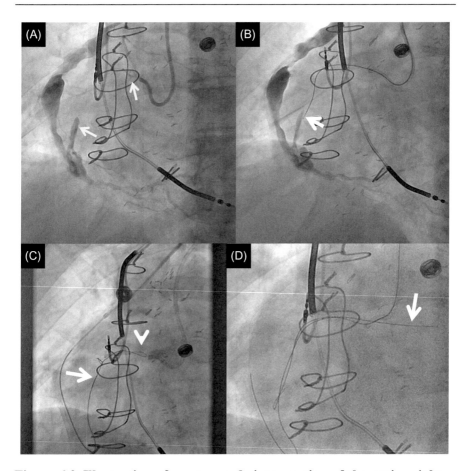

Figure 6.2 Illustration of a retrograde intervention of the native right coronary artery (RCA) (arrows, A) through a degenerated and aneurysmal SVG. After a failed antegrade attempt for CTO crossing (arrow, B), a guidewire was advanced retrogradely into the distal RCA via a SVG with support of a Venture catheter (arrow, C). A "knuckle" (arrowhead, C) was formed on the retrograde guidewire and advanced toward the proximal RCA. After inflation of a 3.0-mm antegrade balloon in the proximal RCA, a Confianza Pro 12 guidewire (arrow, D) was advanced retrogradely into the aorta (reverse CART technique). The guidewire was snared and externalized through a JR4 guide catheter (E), followed by antegrade delivery of drug-eluting stents over the externalized guidewire and restoration of the RCA patency (F).
Source: Reproduced with permission from Ref. 1.

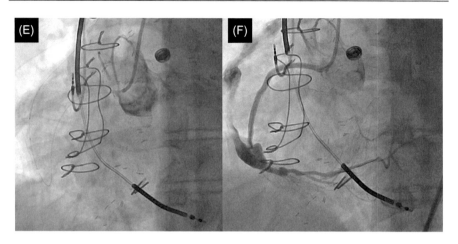

Figure 6.2 (Continued)

Wiring of septal collaterals (Figures 6.3 and 6.4)[6] is preferred over wiring of epicardial collaterals because septal collaterals are usually multiple and are not very tortuous. Injury or perforation of a septal collateral is less likely to cause acute myocardial infarction, myocardial hematoma,[9] or tamponade[25] compared to perforation of an epicardial collateral. Use of epicardial collaterals may be safer in patients with prior coronary bypass graft surgery, as the adhesions may protect against tamponade in case of perforation. However, epicardial hematomas causing cardiac chamber compression[26] and tamponade[23] have been reported. Detailed descriptions of techniques that can stop the bleeding after epicardial collateral perforation are presented in Chapter 12.

Selecting the shorter collateral is preferred because (i) it provides better support and (ii) minimizes the risk of not being able to reach the target lesion. However, if a septal collateral enters the vessel close to the distal cap, there may not be enough space to allow for delivery of a wire and a microcatheter distal to the CTO; using a collateral that enters the vessel more distally is preferred in such cases. Collaterals with corkscrew morphology and >90° angle with the recipient vessel may be challenging or impossible to wire,[12] whereas non-tortuous, large collaterals (CC1 or CC2 by the Werner classification[27] as described in Section 3.3.2) are the easiest to wire.

It is generally easier to advance a wire through a septal collateral from the LAD to the RCA compared from the RCA to the LAD, because

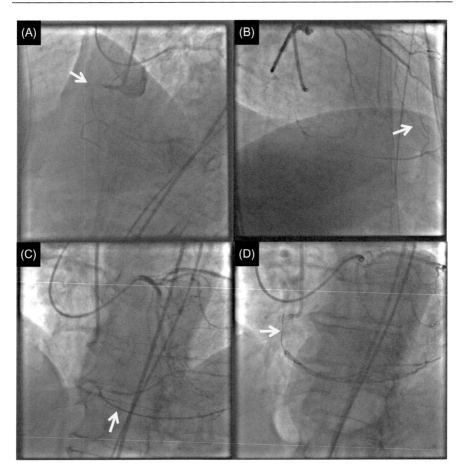

Figure 6.3 Illustration of retrograde intervention with the "just marker" technique (described in detail in Step 7.3 of this chapter). A proximal RCA CTO (arrow, A) could not be crossed antegradely. Left main injection demonstrated a septal collateral branch (arrow, B) that was successfully crossed with a Fielder FC guidewire (arrow, C), which was then advanced to the occlusion site (arrow, D). Using the retrograde wire as a marker, a Confianza Pro 12 wire was advanced antegradely through the CTO (arrow, E), followed by successful stenting of the RCA (F).
Source: Reproduced with permission from Ref. 1.

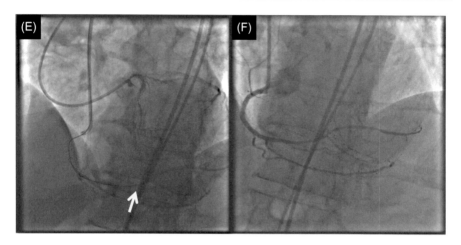

Figure 6.3 (Continued)

the RCA end of the septal collaterals usually has more tortuosity (Figure 6.4B and C).[19]

Finally, **epicardial collaterals** (Figure 6.5) are the least preferred for retrograde CTO PCI,[7] because they are usually more tortuous than septal collaterals[12,13] and their perforation could lead to rapid tamponade, especially in patients with intact pericardium. Moreover, if epicardial collaterals are the only source of collateral blood flow and they become occluded during CTO PCI, acute ischemia (causing bradycardia and/or hypotension in addition to angina) and myocardial infarction may occur. Despite these limitations, with increasing experience and improvements in retrograde equipment (wires and microcatheters), the use of epicardial collaterals has been increasing.

"Invisible" collaterals

Some patients may only appear to have epicardial collaterals, but if those collaterals become occluded, then septal collaterals may also appear (recruitable collaterals). Selective injection, the so-called "tip injection," of the septal perforator branches (through an over-the-wire balloon or through a microcatheter) may also allow visualization of previously "invisible" collaterals. Another option for crossing invisible septal collaterals is with the "surfing" technique (chapter 6, step 4), in which septal collaterals are probed and crossed without contrast injection. This technique increases the success rates of collateral crossing, but has the limitation

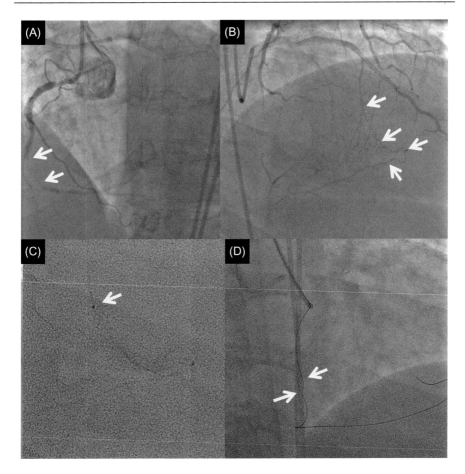

Figure 6.4 Illustration of retrograde intervention with wire externalization. Antegrade crossing attempts of a mid RCA CTO (arrows, A) failed due to the presence of a large side branch at the occlusion site. Injection of the left main demonstrated a large, tortuous septal collateral branch (arrows, B) filling the RCA. Selective injection through a Finecross catheter (arrow, C) highlighted the collateral vessel course. Kissing wire attempts after retrograde and antegrade wires (arrows, D) subintimal advancement in the mid RCA failed. After retrograde puncture with the wire, IVUS (arrow, E) demonstrated that the retrograde wire was located in the proximal true lumen (arrow, F). The retrograde guidewire was trapped into the antegrade guide (arrowhead, G) followed by retrograde balloon dilation (arrows, G) of the CTO. After externalization of the retrograde guidewire a balloon was advanced antegradely (arrow, H), while a retrograde balloon (arrowhead, H) covered the intraseptal portion of the wire. After implantation of multiple drug-eluting stents the RCA patency was restored (I).
Source: Reproduced with permission from Ref. 1.

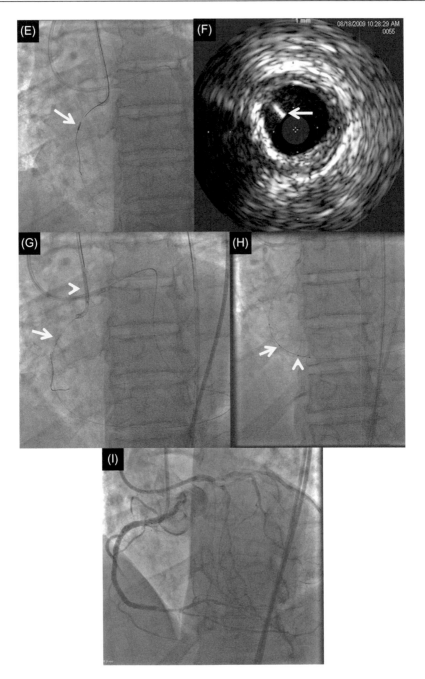

Figure 6.4 (Continued)

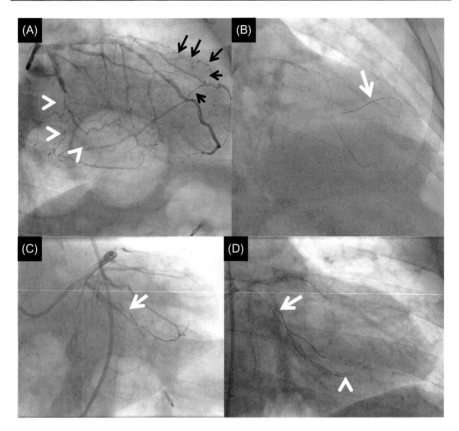

**Figure 6.5 Example of retrograde CTO PCI via an epicardial
collateral.** Coronary angiography demonstrating a CTO of the second
obtuse marginal branch (arrowheads, A), which was filing via an epicardial
collateral from the second diagonal branch (arrows, A). The epicardial
collateral was successfully wired with a Fielder FC wire (arrow, B) through
a Finecross catheter. The retrograde guidewire formed a knuckle (arrow, C)
and was advanced retrogradely in the subintimal space proximal to the
occlusion. After failure of the CART and reverse CART technique, the
antegrade guidewire formed a knuckle and was advanced parallel to the
retrograde guidewire into the subintimal space distal to the occlusion
(arrowhead, D). The retrograde guidewire knuckle is shown by an arrow in
(D). Re-entry into the true lumen distal to the occlusion was achieved with
a Stingray wire (arrowhead, E) through a Stingray balloon (arrow, E).
Stenting restored the patency of the second obtuse marginal branch (F).
Source: Reproduced with permission from Ref. 28.

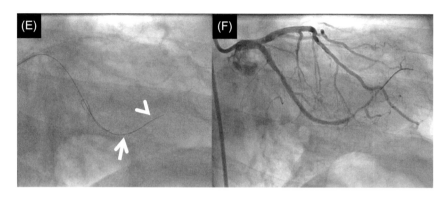

Figure 6.5 (Continued)

that sometimes the collaterals are too small to be tracked by the currently available microcatheters.

Rarely, collateral vessels may not be apparent during diagnostic angiography. For example, an isolated conus branch can occasionally supply collaterals to an occluded LAD territory and has been used for retrograde PCI of such lesions.[29]

Step 3 Getting to the Collateral

Goal: Advance a wire and microcatheter into the target collateral vessel.

How?

— Use a workhorse guidewire to minimize the risk for proximal vessel injury.
— Large, double bends on the workhorse guidewire are often needed to get to the collateral (Figure 6.6). After microcatheter advancement, the wire is exchanged for a collateral crossing guidewire with a small distal bend.
— For collaterals with an acute takeoff from the parent vessel consider using the Venture catheter (Figure 6.7) or an angulated microcatheter (such as the angulated Prowler and Supercross) or the Crusade double lumen catheter (not currently available in the United States) to enter the collateral.

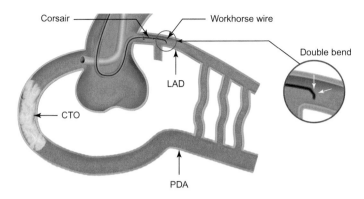

Figure 6.6 Illustration of double bend wire shaping for entering a septal collateral.

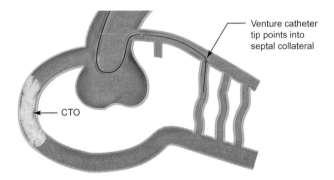

Figure 6.7 Illustration of septal collateral branch wiring using a Venture catheter.

- **Caution**: Wire trapping for removal of the Venture catheter without losing wire position cannot be performed in <8 Fr guides (due to large profile of the Venture catheter).

What can go wrong?

— Injury (such as dissection) of the donor vessel, while trying to enter the collateral. This can be a catastrophic complication (section 12.1.1.1.1), leading to rapid hemodynamic collapse and requires immediate treatment (usually with stenting). Stenting of proximal vessel lesions should be considered prior to retrograde crossing to minimize the risk of proximal vessel dissection (jailing of a septal collateral usually allows wiring of the collateral branch).

Step 4 Crossing the Collateral with a Guidewire

Goal: Cross the collateral with a guidewire.

How?

The technique varies depending on the type of collateral used (septal, epicardial, or SVG).

4a. Septal Collateral

Once the microcatheter is inserted into the septal collateral (Figure 6.8), there are two techniques for subsequent crossing: "surfing" and "contrast-guided."

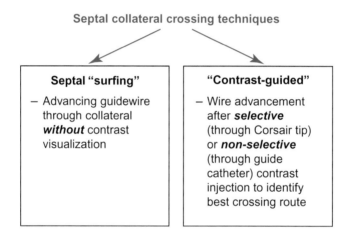

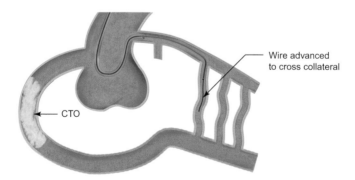

Figure 6.8 Illustration of septal collateral crossing.

Septal "Surfing" Facts

1. Introduced by Dr. George Sianos.
2. The guidewire (Sion is more commonly used currently) is **advanced rapidly** until it either "buckles" or advances into the distal target vessel. If the wire "buckles" it is withdrawn and redirected.
3. Septal surfing can be a very **efficient** crossing method.

Septal Surfing: Tips and Tricks

1. Surfing should **NEVER** be done in epicardial collaterals, because of high risk for perforation.
2. If the wire repeatedly takes the same unsuccessful course, *retract further back* before re-advancing to select alternate route.
3. **Do NOT push hard**—force will increase the risk of collateral injury without increasing crossing success.
4. The odds of successful wiring are usually higher in **proximal**, straighter septals.
5. Septal collaterals usually run straight down in their upper half (LAD side), then bow toward the apex and turn again into the PDA (Figure 6.9).

    Therefore RAO cranial is the best projection for initial wiring, and RAO caudal for entering into the posterior descending artery.

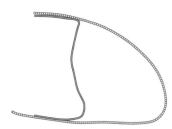

Figure 6.9 RAO caudal view of septal collaterals.

"Contrast-Guided" Septal Crossing

1. Use 3-mL luer-lock syringe with 100% contrast.
2. First aspirate until blood enters syringe (to avoid air embolization).
3. Perform cine-angiography while injecting contrast with the 3-mL syringe.
4. Flush microcatheter before re-inserting guidewire (to minimize subsequent "stickiness").
5. If a continuous connection to distal vessel is observed, re-attempt crossing through that connection.
6. Do NOT pan to avoid change in collateral road mapping.
7. Consider right anterior oblique (RAO) caudal projection to evaluate the length and tortuosity of the distal part of the septal collateral. Also left anterior oblique (LAO) projections can be useful if there is limited progress with the RAO views.

What can go wrong?

1. Collateral dissection (in most cases further attempts to cross may be performed via a different collateral).
2. Collateral perforation (which is nearly always benign and only causes localized staining; however, there are reported cases of septal hematoma formation[9] and/or perforation into the pericardium causing tamponade[25]).
3. Guidewire entrapment: To prevent this complication do not allow big (>1.5 mm) and acute (>75°) bends to form at the tip of the guidewire during attempts for retrograde crossing of the septal collateral.[30]

4b. Epicardial Collateral

Epicardial Collateral Crossing Facts

1. Should always be performed using contrast guidance (i.e., no "surfing").
2. Orthogonal injections are important to determine the collateral vessel course.
3. It is safer in patients with prior sternotomy, as pericardial adhesions may prevent pericardial fluid accumulation and tamponade (however, tamponade is still possible in case of perforation).
4. Marked tortuosity and small collateral size reduces the likelihood of successful collateral vessel crossing.

Epicardial Collateral Crossing: Tips and Tricks

1. Perform injection through microcatheter to visualize the collateral vessel course. Be certain that the microcatheter is not "wedged" and inject gently to avoid collateral damage.
2. Advance wire first, then follow with Corsair—never let Corsair advance ahead of guidewire.
3. Microcatheter will "straighten" tortuosity and allow subsequent advancement.
4. Rotate the wire (do not push) in tortuous segments. Crossing may be easier during diastole, when the angle between collateral turns is wider (Figure 6.10).
5. Once the wire reaches the distal true lumen it is advanced to the distal cap before following with the microcatheter.

What can go wrong?

1. Collateral dissection (in most cases further attempts to cross can be performed via a different collateral).
2. Collateral perforation that can cause tamponade (tamponade is less likely to occur in patients with prior coronary artery bypass graft surgery).

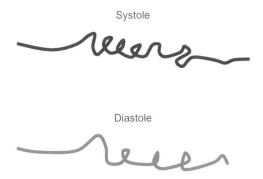

Systole

Diastole

Figure 6.10 Illustration of changes in epicardial collateral channel angulation during the cardiac cycle. In tortuous epicardial channels, wire crossing through the spiraling segments is the key to success. When the tip gets caught in the curve, quick torque of the wire tends to slide a little on a wider angle in diastole. Therefore, timely torqueing is necessary to go through the spiral segment of the channel.

3. Guidewire entrapment: To prevent this, the operator should not allow a loop or "knuckle" to form at the tip of the guidewire during attempts for retrograde crossing of the septal collateral.[30]

4. Ischemia of the myocardium supplied by the collateral, especially if there are no other collaterals supplying the same territory.

4c. Bypass Graft

Bypass Grafts for Retrograde CTO PCI: Tips and Tricks

1. Both arterial grafts and SVGs (either patent or occluded) can be used.

2. There is a risk for perforation and distal embolization (with either patent or occluded SVGs).

3. Internal-mammary artery (IMA) bypass grafts are the least preferred bypass grafts for retrograde wiring, because insertion of equipment in the graft could result in pseudolesion formation and even antegrade flow cessation[31] and because injury of the IMA graft might have catastrophic consequences.

4. One of the major challenges of retrograde wiring through bypass grafts is navigating severe angulation at the distal anastomosis. This can be overcome by several techniques, such as using:

    a. hydrophilic guidewires and preshaped microcatheters, such as the Prowler microcatheters,[32]

    b. the reversed guidewire technique,[33,34]

    c. the Venture deflectable tip catheter,[35,36] or

    d. a magnetically enabled guidewire, such as the Titan or Pegasus wires if a magnetic navigation system is available.[1]

5. After a native coronary CTO is recanalized, coiling of the SVG may be considered (to minimize risk for subsequent distal embolization) although this approach is controversial.

Step 5 Confirm Guidewire Position Within the Distal True Lumen

Goal: Confirm that the retrograde guidewire has crossed through the collateral into the distal true lumen.

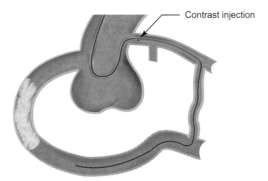

Contrast injection

Figure 6.11 Illustration of distal true lumen positioning of the retrograde guidewire, which is an imperative step before advancing the microcatheter through the collateral.

How?

By injecting contrast through the retrograde guide catheter (Figures 6.11 and 6.12).

Distal Wire Position Confirmation

— Angiographic confirmation of distal guidewire position should always be done **before** advancing the Corsair through the collateral (to prevent collateral rupture if the wire has exited the vessel) (Figure 6.12A).
— Possible wire positions
  • Septum (no crossing achieved).
  • Distal true lumen.
  • Cavity (suspected if the wire starts making large back-and-forth movements).
  • Pericardium.
  • Non-septal collateral (occasionally a collateral may appear to be a septal in one projection but may in reality be epicardial; such collaterals have higher risk of rupture; a classic example is an acute marginal collateral supplying the RCA from the distal LAD artery). Obtaining an orthogonal view can help clarify the collateral type and location.

(A)

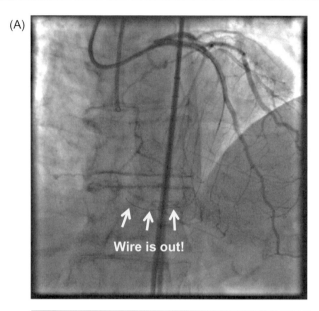

(B)

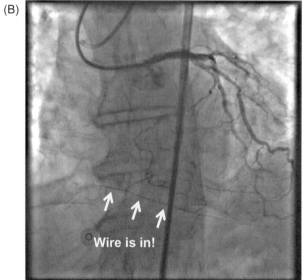

Figure 6.12 Example of extraluminal retrograde guidewire position (A). The wire was repositioned achieving intraluminal position (B). (A) Wire located outside the distal true lumen—the Corsair microcatheter should not be advanced with the guidewire in this position. (B) Wire located inside the distal true lumen—the Corsair microcatheter can now be advanced over the wire.

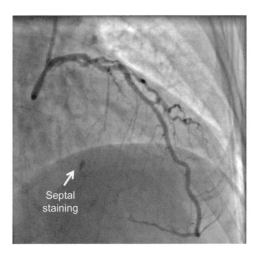

Figure 6.13 Example of septal staining after retrograde septal wiring attempts.

- The Corsair should be advanced only if the guidewire is located into the distal true lumen. In all other cases, the wire should be retracted and redirected.
- Septal staining is almost always benign and does not cause tamponade (but can cause cardiac biomarker elevation) (Figure 6.13).

Step 6 Crossing the Collateral with the Microcatheter

Goal: To advance the microcatheter into the distal true lumen.

How?

After distal true lumen guidewire position is confirmed, the guidewire is advanced as far as possible close to the distal CTO cap (or deeply in another distal branch, such as the posterolateral branch) to provide sufficient backup for retrograde microcatheter advancement (Figure 6.14).

What to do if the microcatheter will not advance through the collateral.

1. Rapid clockwise and counterclockwise rotation of the microcatheter, using both hands.

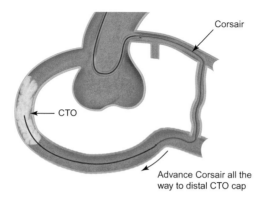

Figure 6.14 Advancing the microcatheter into the distal true lumen.

2. Increase retrograde guide catheter support, either with active support (forward push of left-sided guides or clockwise rotation of right-sided guides) or by using a side-branch anchor technique or a guide catheter extension, such as the Guideliner and Guidezilla (Section 3.6).
3. Dilate collateral (septal only — never dilate an epicardial collateral) with a small (1.20—1.5 mm) balloon at low pressure (2—4 atm).
4. Try another microcatheter (sometimes the Corsair can become "sticky" with prolonged use; using a new Corsair catheter may be successful).
5. If the Corsair microcatheter fails to cross, replace with a Finecross microcatheter as its external diameter is smaller (2.6 versus 1.8 Fr, respectively).
6. If the retrograde guidewire is located adjacent to an antegrade subintimal guidewire, the retrograde guidewire can be anchored by inflating a balloon over the antegrade guidewire. Anchoring can provide enough support to advance the microcatheter through the collateral.

Alternatively, if the microcatheter cannot cross the septal collateral:

1. Attempt to cross the CTO with the retrograde guidewire (more likely to be successful in short, non-calcified occlusions).
2. Use the retrograde guidewire as "just marker" for antegrade crossing.
3. Try to use another collateral.

What can go wrong?

1. Ischemia can occur, if most or all of the CTO target vessel perfusion comes from the wired collateral. This is most likely to occur with epicardial collaterals, as there are usually many septal collaterals. Mild chest discomfort is, however, common during retrograde crossing.

2. Retrograde guide position loss, usually with excessive advancement of the retrograde microcatheter in spite of resistance. To prevent this, careful attention should be paid to the retrograde guide position.
3. Injury of the donor vessel (especially if there is excessive back-and-forth movement of the retrograde guide catheter).
4. Donor vessel thrombosis (particularly in long retrograde cases and if the donor vessel is diseased). To avoid this, the ACT should be maintained at >350 s.

Step 7 Crossing the CTO

Goal: Cross the CTO with a guidewire.

How?

Once the collateral branch has been successfully wired and the retrograde microcatheter advanced to the distal cap, there are three ways to cross the lesion:[1]

1. Retrograde crossing of the CTO into the proximal true lumen (retrograde "true lumen puncture" or "true to true").
2. Retrograde dissection/re-entry techniques.
3. Antegrade crossing of the CTO (using the "kissing wire" or the "just marker" technique).

All techniques require excellent guide support that can be achieved using the techniques described in Section 3.6.[37]

6.5   Retrograde True Lumen Puncture

Retrograde true lumen puncture can be achieved in approximately 20–40% of retrograde CTO PCIs (Figures 6.4 and 6.15).[12]

The wire that crossed the collateral is advanced to the CTO distal cap, followed by advancement of the microcatheter or over-the-wire balloon for additional support. The CTO is then crossed from the distal into the proximal true lumen, either with the same guidewire (as the distal CTO cap may be softer and more tapered than the proximal cap) or with a stiffer guidewire.[1]

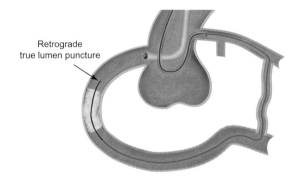

Retrograde
true lumen puncture

Figure 6.15 Illustration of retrograde true lumen puncture.

Several maneuvers can be used to enhance the chance of crossing, such as inflating a retrograde balloon for more support (coaxial anchor) and using stiffer, tapered-tip, and/or hydrophilic wires. However, some argue that use of highly penetrating guidewires (such as the Confianza Pro 12 guidewire) should be avoided because if retrograde perforation occurs it may be difficult to control. Antegrade intravascular ultrasonography (IVUS) can also facilitate directing the retrograde guidewire into the proximal true lumen (Figure 6.4F).[38,39]

6.6   Retrograde Dissection/Re-entry

If during manipulation of the antegrade, retrograde, or both guidewires the CTO subintimal space is entered, re-entry into the true lumen and CTO crossing can be achieved by two techniques (Figure 6.16):[1,2]

a. Inflating a balloon over the retrograde guidewire, followed by advancement of the antegrade guidewire into the distal true lumen (controlled antegrade and retrograde tracking and dissection—CART).[5]
b. Inflating a balloon over the antegrade guidewire, followed by advancement of the retrograde guidewire into the proximal true lumen (reverse CART).

Several variations of the CART techniques have been reported, such as the IVUS-guided CART,[13] the Guideliner-assisted CART, the "stent reverse CART," and the "confluent balloon"[40] technique.

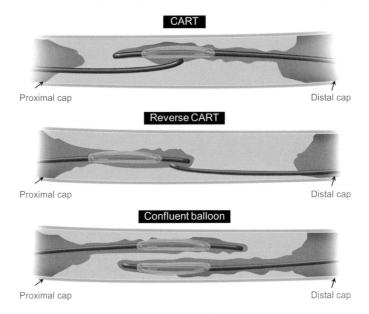

Figure 6.16 Illustration of the retrograde dissection re-entry techniques.

6.6.1 CART Technique

First described by Katoh et al. in 2006,[5] the CART technique is based on the principle of creating a subintimal space (ideally confined to the CTO segment) that is known to communicate with the true lumen (Figures 6.16 and 6.17). The subintimal space is enlarged by inflating a balloon inserted over the retrograde wire.[5] While the balloon is being deflated, the contralateral wire is directed toward the balloon, crossing the lesion and entering the path taken by the balloon and wire. Usually 2.5−3.0 mm diameter balloons are used for the CART technique. After CTO crossing with an antegrade guidewire, balloon angioplasty and stenting is performed in a standard manner.

This technique is often limited by the ability of the balloon to cross the collateral vessel. In the initial period, balloon dilation of the septal collaterals was mandatory. In modern days use of the Corsair catheter allows for (rapid-exchange or over-the-wire) balloon crossing without further channel dilation. However, the need for retrograde balloon advancement has been largely replaced by the reverse CART technique and is only used in cases in which the retrograde equipment is

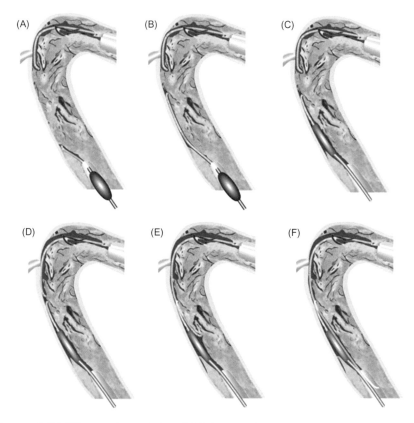

Figure 6.17 Illustration of the CART technique. Step-by-step illustration of the controlled antegrade and retrograde tracking and dissection technique. The retrograde guidewire reaches the distal CTO cap (A) and is advanced into the CTO subintimal space (B). A balloon is advanced over the retrograde guidewire into the subintimal space (C) where it is inflated (D), enabling advancement of the antegrade guidewire into the space created by the balloon (E), which communicates with the distal true lumen (F). *Source*: Reproduced with permission from HMP Communications.[5]

not long enough to reach the antegrade guiding catheter (mainly in patients with long epicardial connections and very enlarged hearts).

6.6.2   Reverse CART Technique

The reverse CART technique is similar to the CART technique, with the difference that the balloon is inflated over the antegrade guidewire, creating a space into which the retrograde guidewire is advanced (Figure 6.16). The most common causes of CART and reverse CART failure are related to inability to connect the different spaces (e.g., true lumen in one and subintimal in the other) and use of undersized balloons. Balloon sizing can be facilitated using IVUS, which allows measurement of the media-to-media dimensions. With the development of the Corsair catheter, the reverse CART technique has largely supplanted the CART technique for CTO crossing (antegrade wire passage is less predictable with CART and externalization cannot be performed with CART).[41]

After retrograde guidewire crossing, **wire externalization is performed in most cases** (Step 8, described below). Other treatment options include antegrade wiring and retrograde stent delivery.

6.6.2.1 Antegrade Wiring

One way to complete the CTO PCI after retrograde wire crossing is to perform balloon angioplasty of the CTO segment using a balloon advanced over the retrograde guidewire to create a lumen through the CTO followed by antegrade wire crossing and PCI. Retrograde balloon angioplasty can be facilitated by advancing the retrograde wire far into the aorta, or, if possible, into the antegrade guide where it can be "trapped" with an antegrade balloon inflated at 10−15 atm (Figure 6.4G). Other support techniques can improve the retrograde deliverability of equipment, such as the double balloon anchoring technique, in which the retrograde wire in anchored into the antegrade guide, and the retrograde guide is anchored in the donor vessel ostium by inflating a balloon in a small vessel side branch.[42]

Other strategies used to enable antegrade wiring after retrograde crossing include:

1. The "antegrade microcatheter probing technique" in which the retrograde microcatheter is advanced into the antegrade guide catheter, followed by removal of the retrograde guidewire and intubation of the microcatheter with an antegrade wire.[43]
2. The "bridge or rendezvous method" in which the retrograde microcatheter is inserted into the antegrade guide and aligned with an antegrade microcatheter allowing insertion of an antegrade guidewire distal to the CTO.[38,44]

3. The "reverse wire trapping technique" that involves snaring of the retrograde guidewire followed by withdrawal of the retrograde guidewire pulling the antegrade snare through the CTO into the distal true lumen.[45]

4. Externalization of the wire (as described in Step 8) followed by antegrade insertion of a microcatheter, over which an antegrade wire is inserted.[46] The advantage of all these techniques is that they minimize retrograde guidewire and balloon manipulations after retrograde crossing but wiring a microcatheter can be challenging. Moreover, wire externalization can provide superior support for antegrade equipment delivery.

After antegrade wire crossing, antegrade crossing with balloons and stents can be challenging. Reverse anchoring (anchoring the antegrade wire by inflation of a retrograde balloon) can provide strong backup support for antegrade equipment delivery.[43,47]

If an antegrade wire cannot cross the CTO in spite of multiple retrograde balloon inflations, different strategies can be used, such as (1) externalization of the retrograde wire (Step 8)[17] or (2) retrograde delivery of stents in selected cases.

6.6.2.2   Retrograde Delivery of Stents

This technique is performed extremely rarely due to high risk for stent loss or entrapment, but retrograde stent delivery has been reported through both septal[48] and epicardial[49] collaterals. It requires adequate predilation of the collateral to minimize the risk of injury and stent entrapment or dislodgement.[50] After completion of the intervention, the donor artery is imaged again to ascertain that no complication has occurred.

6.6.3   Variations of the Reverse CART Technique

Several modifications of the reverse CART technique have been developed:[1,2] Rathore et al. proposed the **IVUS-guided CART** technique to allow more precise sizing of the balloon (to maximize the space created for re-entry without risking vessel rupture) and to determine whether significant recoil occurs after ballooning (in which cases repeat balloon inflations are performed with a larger balloon or a snare is inserted into the subintimal dissection plane to keep it open) (Figure 6.18).[13] IVUS also allows visualization of the

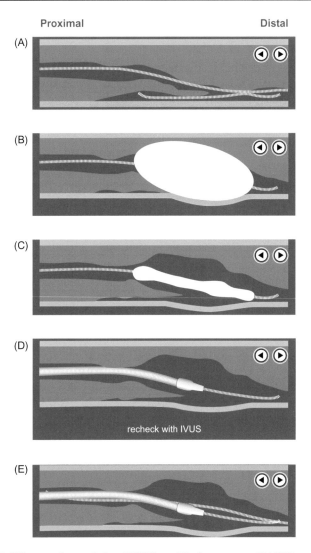

Figure 6.18 Illustration of the IVUS-guided reverse CART technique. (A) shows both antegrade and retrograde guidewire in the subintimal space. (B and C) demonstrate dilation of subintimal space with balloon on the antegrade wire to create a connection. (D) shows checking with IVUS for the location of subintimal space, and (E) illustrates retrograde wire passage from the subintimal space into the antegrade true lumen via a connection made by the antegrade balloon under IVUS guidance.
Source: Reproduced with permission from Ref. 13.

retrograde wire as it enters the enlarged subintimal space that communicates with the true lumen.

Wu et al.[39] proposed a modification of the reverse CART technique, in which the antegrade balloon remains inflated during retrograde crossing attempts and is "**punctured**" by the retrograde guidewire, which is then advanced while the punctured antegrade balloon is retracted under fluoroscopy.

Occasionally, a **guide catheter extension** (Guideliner or Guidezilla) can be advanced over the antegrade guidewire to form a proximal target for the retrograde guidewire and facilitate entry into the guide catheter.

In the "**stent reverse CART**" technique, a stent is placed in the proximal true lumen into the subintimal space to facilitate retrograde wiring into the stent.

In another variation entitled "**confluent balloon technique**," both antegrade and retrograde balloons are inflated simultaneously in a kissing fashion to cause the subintimal space to become confluent, allowing wire passage through the CTO (Figure 6.19).[40]

Contrast injections through the guide should not be performed after any attempts for reverse CART, since this will enlarge and extend the localized dissection downstream. To prevent this, the injection syringe can be disconnected from the manifold, as illustrated in Figure 5.7).

What can go wrong?

a. As with all dissection strategies (antegrade and retrograde), side branches at the area of dissection may become occluded, with consequences dependent on the size of the supplied territory (see Section 12.1.1.1.3).
b. Vessel perforation, if the subintimal balloon is oversized (although most commonly it is undersized). IVUS can help optimize the subintimal balloon size.

6.7 Antegrade Crossing

"**Just marker**" (Figure 6.20) is the simplest (but least reliable) form of the retrograde technique: The retrograde wire is advanced to the distal cap and acts as a marker of the distal true lumen, serving as a

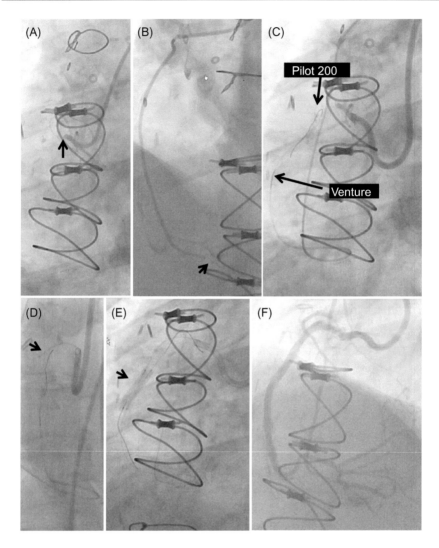

Figure 6.19 Illustration of the "confluent balloon" technique. CTO of the proximal RCA (arrow, A) with filling of the right posterior descending artery via a diffusely diseased SVG with a distal anastomotic lesion (arrow, B). Using a Venture catheter and a Pilot 200 wire formed into a knuckle (arrow, C), the CTO was crossed subintimally. A CrossBoss catheter was used for antegrade crossing (arrow, D), followed by inflation of two 2.5-mm balloons, one advanced over the antegrade and the other advanced over the retrograde guidewire (arrow, E) ("confluent balloon" technique). The CTO was successfully crossed with an excellent result after stent implantation (F).
Source: Reproduced with permission from Ref. 51.

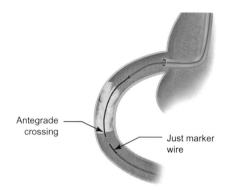

Antegrade crossing

Just marker wire

Figure 6.20 Illustration of the "just marker" technique.

target for the antegrade wire.[8,37] This allows continuous visualization of where the distal true lumen is located, without contrast injections.

"Kissing wire" entails manipulation of both the antegrade and the retrograde wires in the CTO until the ends of the wires meet; the antegrade wire then follows the channel made by the retrograde wire into the true lumen of the distal vessel.[1,37]

Step 8 Wire Externalization

Goal: To externalize the retrograde guidewire, in order to use it as rail to advance balloons and stents in an antegrade direction, followed by safe removal of the externalized equipment.

This step is only applicable to cases in which the CTO is crossed in the retrograde direction (retrograde true lumen puncture and reverse CART). If the CTO is crossed in the antegrade direction this step is not feasible or required.

How?

Two options are available for retrograde wire externalization depending on whether the retrograde guidewire enters the antegrade guide or not: (a) wiring the antegrade guide and (b) snaring. **Wiring the antegrade guide** is simpler and preferable and may be facilitated by advancing a guide catheter extension (such as Guideliner or Guidezilla) into the antegrade vessel. This may not always be possible, especially in the following circumstances:

1. Aortoostial CTOs.
2. Large vessel caliber.
3. Non-coaxial guide positioning.

Option A. Retrograde guidewire enters into the antegrade guide catheter

Wiring the antegrade guide catheter with the retrograde guidewire is the simplest technique to externalize a guidewire and should be the first choice whenever possible (Figure 6.21).

1. After the retrograde wire (that crossed the CTO) enters the antegrade guide, a trapping balloon is inflated within the antegrade guide next to the wire to facilitate advancement of the retrograde microcatheter into the antegrade guide catheter (Figure 6.22A).
2. The retrograde guidewire is removed, while the retrograde microcatheter remains within the antegrade guide catheter (Figure 6.22B).

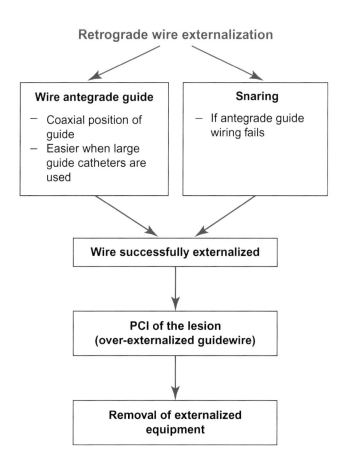

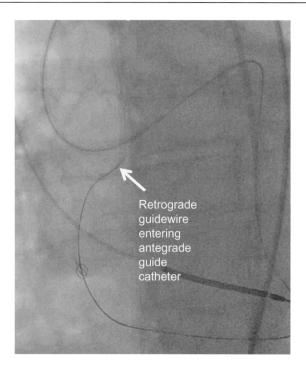

Retrograde
guidewire
entering
antegrade
guide
catheter

Figure 6.21 Example or retrograde wire entering the antegrade guide catheter.

3. The microcatheter is flushed with Rotaglide (to reduce friction and facilitate advancement of the externalization wire) (Figure 6.22C).
4. The wire to be externalized (Viper 335 or R350) is inserted and pushed through the microcatheter (Figure 6.22D).
5. The antegrade Y-connector is disconnected from the guide catheter and a finger is placed over the antegrade guide catheter hub, until the retrograde guidewire is felt "tapping" on the finger (Figure 6.22E).
6. A wire introducer is inserted through the antegrade Y-connector and the retrograde guidewire tip is threaded through the introducer (Figure 6.22F).
7. The antegrade Y-connector is reconnected to the guide catheter hub, **without flushing** (to avoid an antegrade hydraulic dissection) (Figure 6.22G).
8. The retrograde guidewire is pushed until 20–30 cm have exited through the Y-connector.
9. If the tip of the externalized guidewire is damaged, it can be cut off to facilitate loading of balloons/stents or other equipment.

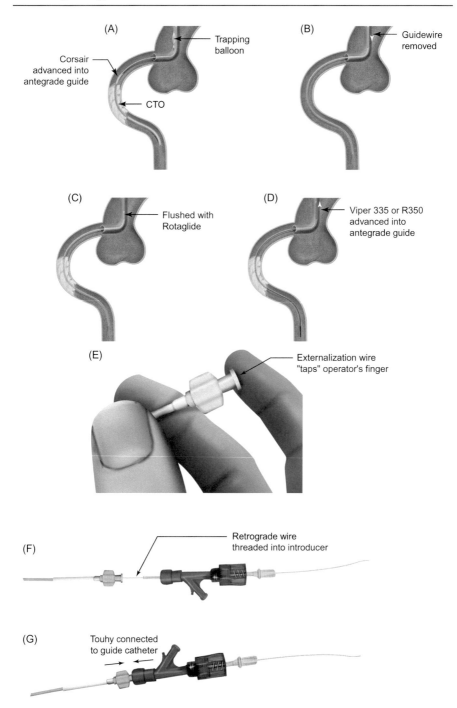

Figure 6.22 Step-by-step illustration of the retrograde wire externalization technique.

Option B. Snaring the retrograde guidewire

If wiring the antegrade guide catheter with the retrograde wire fails, then wire snaring can be performed (as described in Section 2.6.1). If the retrograde microcatheter successfully crossed the lesion into the aorta, then an externalization wire (Viper 335, R350, RG3) can be advanced through it and snared. If not, then the wire used for retrograde lesion crossing can be externalized and if it is not long enough it can then be exchanged for a long externalization wire.

1. Snare preparation (illustrated in Section 2.6.1).
   - Of the commercially available snares, the 27−45 or 18−30 mm En Snare has three loops facilitating capture of the retrograde guidewire and is preferred to single loop snares, such as the Microvena Amplatz Goose Neck snares and microsnares and the Micro Elite snare.
   - The snare is removed from the package and pulled back into the snare introducer.
   - The snare delivery catheter is discarded (the guide catheter is used for snare delivery).
   - The snare is inserted into antegrade guide by inserting the introducer through the Y-connector (a Co-pilot or a Guardian is preferred to minimize bleeding).
   - If snaring is performed through a guide for the right coronary artery, it is preferable to use a JR4 guide instead of an Amplatz guide (which is used for most antegrade CTO attempts), as the JR4 guide catheter poses less risk for ostial RCA dissection.
2. The snare is advanced out of antegrade guide and opened (Figure 6.23A).
3. The retrograde guidewire is advanced through the snare (Figure 6.23B). It is preferable to snare the guidewire you plan to externalize (Viper, RG3, or R350). This is dependent on getting the Corsair into the aorta. The radiopaque portion of these wires is snared, followed by careful sweep into the antegrade guide catheter.

   If it is not possible to advance the Corsair through the CTO and into the aorta, a standard length wire may need to be snared. More care must be taken when these wires are snared to avoid fracture or unraveling of the distal part of the guidewire. The ideal snaring location is immediately proximal to the radiopaque portion of the wire.
4. The snare is pulled back capturing the retrograde guidewire (arrow, Figure 6.23C).

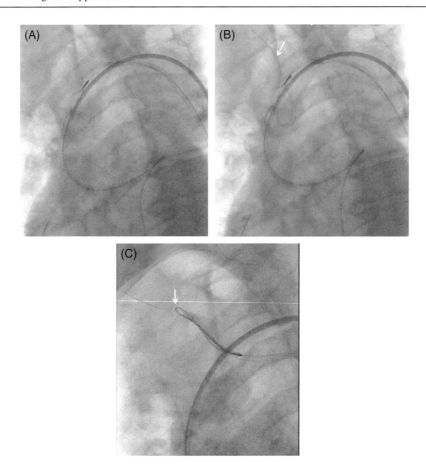

Figure 6.23 Illustration of snaring a retrograde guidewire. (A) Illustration of a three-loop snare advanced through the guide catheter and deployed in the ascending aorta. (B) The retrograde guidewire (arrow) is advanced through the snare. (C) Snare withdrawal capturing the retrograde guidewire.

What can go wrong?

    a. Snaring the distal flexible portion of the retrograde wire can result in wire fracture,[45,52] although this is very unlikely with currently used externalization wires, such as the Viper and R350.

    b. The snared wire may unravel (which is why snaring should be performed under continuous fluoroscopic observation).

5. The retrograde guidewire is pushed through the retrograde microcatheter (while applying gentle traction on the snare) until it exits from the antegrade guide Y-connector (Figure 6.24).

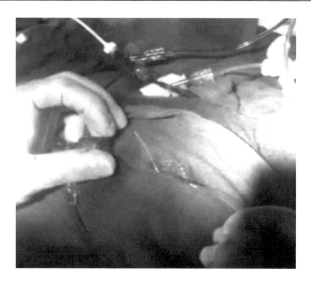

Figure 6.24 Example of snared retrograde guidewire exiting from the antegrade guide Y-connector.

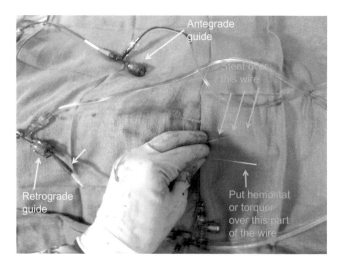

Figure 6.25 Example of an externalized guidewire that is ready for balloon and stent delivery.

The deformed wire tip is then cut to facilitate loading of equipment over the externalized portion of the guidewire.

6. Preparing for angioplasty and stenting.

   1. The microcatheter is retracted distal to the CTO (but continues to cover the portion of the externalized guidewire that is coursing within the collateral vessel to prevent collateral injury).
   2. A torquer or hemostat is attached to the proximal end of the externalized guidewire (to reduce the risk for inadvertent withdrawal of the wire into the microcatheter) (Figure 6.25).

Step 9 Treatment of the CTO

After the retrograde guidewire has been successfully externalized, balloon angioplasty and stenting can be performed using rapid-exchange equipment, followed by removal of the externalized guidewire.

9a. Balloon Angioplasty and Stenting

- The externalized guidewire provides outstanding support, allowing easy delivery of virtually any device.
- The tip of the antegrade balloon/catheters should never be allowed to "meet" with the tip of the retrograde microcatheter/balloon on the same guidewire, because "interlocking" can occur, resulting in equipment entrapment that may require surgery for removal (see Section 12.1.1.1.3).

9b. Externalized Guidewire Removal

1. Once stenting of the CTO is completed (Figure 6.26A), the retrograde wire needs to be removed in a safe manner.
2. The retrograde microcatheter is advanced back into the antegrade guide (through the recently deployed stents, Figure 6.26B), unless resistance is encountered.
3. Both guide catheters are disengaged (Figure 6.26C) (to minimize the risk for the guides getting "sucked into" the coronary ostia, potentially causing dissection).
   - The antegrade guide is disengaged by pushing the externalized guidewire.
   - The retrograde guide is disengaged by fixing the microcatheter and using it as rail for guide retraction.
4. The retrograde guidewire is withdrawn (Figure 6.26D).

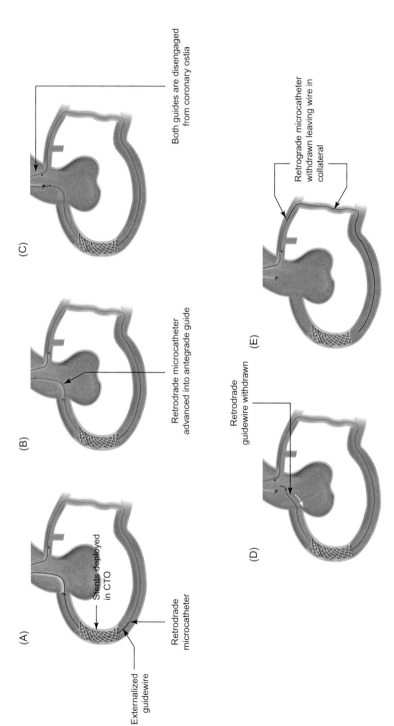

(A)

Externalized
guidewire

Stents deployed
in CTO

Retrodrade
microcatheter

(B)

Retrodrade microcatheter
advanced into antegrade guide

(C)

Both guides are disengaged
from coronary ostia

(D)

Retrodrade
guidewire withdrawn

(E)

Retrograde microcatheter
withdrawn leaving wire in
collateral

Figure 6.26 Illustration of the steps involved with removal of the externalized guidewire.

5. The retrograde microcatheter is withdrawn into the donor vessel leaving the retrograde guidewire through the collateral (Figure 6.26E).
6. Contrast is injected via the retrograde guide to ensure that no injury (perforation of rupture) of the collateral vessel has occurred. If injury is detected, the microcatheter (or a new microcatheter) can be re-advanced over the retrograde guidewire to cover the collateral channel perforation and possibly deliver coils or thrombin.
7. If no collateral vessel injury is detected, the guidewire is removed after re-advancing the microcatheter over the guidewire to minimize the risk for injury, especially in tortuous epicardial collaterals.

What can go wrong?

1. Collateral dissection: The wire crossing the collateral should always be covered with a microcatheter or over-the-wire balloon to minimize the risk for collateral vessel injury.
2. Dissection of the target vessel ostia (beware of guide catheter movement during externalization; the externalized guidewire should be pushed out rather than pulled).
3. Collateral perforation: Collateral perforation can occur during attempts to cross the collateral or during equipment delivery.
4. Equipment entrapment: The antegrade balloon/stents should not meet the retrograde microcatheter or balloon to minimize the risk of catheter "interlocking" and entrapment.

6.8   Special Retrograde CTO PCI Scenarios

6.8.1   Ipsilateral Collateral

In patients with ipsilateral collaterals (such as septal collaterals from the proximal into the distal LAD (Figure 6.27), or diagonal or obtuse marginal left-to-left collaterals), dual injection may not be required.[53,54]

a. A special challenge with ipsilateral collaterals is that the retrograde wire has to take a fairly sharp turn to return into the proximal vessel, which can lead to kinking and difficulty advancing equipment,[54] or, more importantly, to collateral rupture (which occurs more frequently with ipsilateral than contralateral collaterals).
b. If the CTO is successfully wired through the collateral, then a second ipsilateral guide catheter may be beneficial for trapping or externalizing

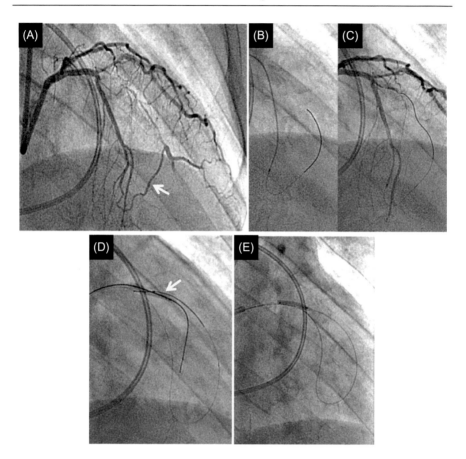

Figure 6.27 Example of retrograde CTO PCI of an LAD artery using the retrograde approach via a septal—septal channel. Coronary angiography demonstrating a mid LAD artery CTO with the distal vessel filling via an ipsilateral septal collateral (arrow, A). Crossing of the ipsilateral collateral was achieved with a Pilot guidewire (B), followed by retrograde crossing into the proximal LAD using the reverse CART technique (C and D). The CTO was predilated (E), followed by antegrade wiring (F) and stenting with an excellent final result (G).
Source: Modified with permission from Ref. 53.

the wire, because if the retrograde wire is inserted into the antegrade guide catheter, equipment delivery is more difficult through the same guide catheter. Equipment delivery is easier using a "ping-pong" technique, in which engagement of the target vessel is alternating between the two guide catheters (Figure 6.28).[55]

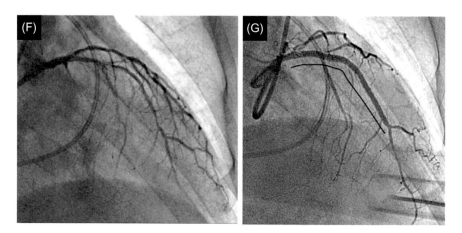

Figure 6.27 (Continued)

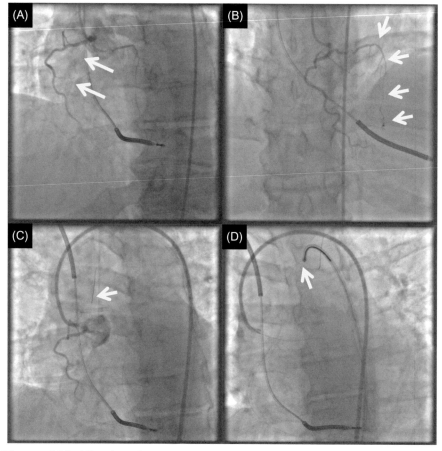

Figure 6.28 (Continued)

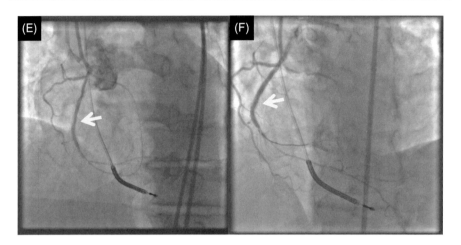

Figure 6.28 (Continued)

6.8.2 Ostial CTOs

In patients with ostial CTOs, antegrade guide engagement may not be feasible; hence, retrograde may be the only possible crossing strategy. In one reported case, retrograde delivery of a stent through a septal collateral was required to treat such a lesion.[48] An alternative treatment strategy would be to snare and externalize the retrograde guidewire followed by antegrade stent delivery.

◀ **Figure 6.28 Example of the "ping-pong" guide catheter technique for retrograde CTO PCI via an ipsilateral collateral.** Coronary angiography demonstrating a proximal RCA CTO due to in-stent restenosis (arrows, A), with an ipsilateral atrial collateral (arrows, B). Retrograde CTO crossing with wire exiting into the aorta (C) followed by successful snaring through a second guide catheter (D) and stenting (E and F) using the two guide catheters in a "ping-pong" fashion.
Source: Reproduced with permission from Ref. 55.

References

1. Brilakis ES, Grantham JA, Thompson CA, et al. The retrograde approach to coronary artery chronic total occlusions: a practical approach. *Catheter Cardiovasc Interv* 2012;**79**:3–19.
2. Joyal D, Thompson CA, Grantham JA, Buller CEH, Rinfret S. The retrograde technique for recanalization of chronic total occlusions: a step-by-step approach. *JACC Cardiovasc Interv* 2012;**5**:1–11.
3. Kahn JK, Hartzler GO. Retrograde coronary angioplasty of isolated arterial segments through saphenous vein bypass grafts. *Cathet Cardiovasc Diagn* 1990;**20**:88–93.
4. Silvestri M, Parikh P, Roquebert PO, Barragan P, Bouvier JL, Comet B. Retrograde left main stenting. *Cathet Cardiovasc Diagn* 1996;**39**:396–9.
5. Surmely JF, Tsuchikane E, Katoh O, et al. New concept for CTO recanalization using controlled antegrade and retrograde subintimal tracking: the CART technique. *J Invasive Cardiol* 2006;**18**:334–8.
6. Ozawa N. A new understanding of chronic total occlusion from a novel PCI technique that involves a retrograde approach to the right coronary artery via a septal branch and passing of the guidewire to a guiding catheter on the other side of the lesion. *Catheter Cardiovasc Interv* 2006;**68**:907–13.
7. Kumar SS, Kaplan B. Chronic total occlusion angioplasty through supplying collaterals. *Catheter Cardiovasc Interv* 2006;**68**:914–6.
8. Niccoli G, Ochiai M, Mazzari MA. A complex case of right coronary artery chronic total occlusion treated by a successful multi-step Japanese approach. *J Invasive Cardiol* 2006;**18**:E230–3.
9. Lin TH, Wu DK, Su HM, et al. Septum hematoma: a complication of retrograde wiring in chronic total occlusion. *Int J Cardiol* 2006;**113**: e64–6.
10. Rosenmann D, Meerkin D, Almagor Y. Retrograde dilatation of chronic total occlusions via collateral vessel in three patients. *Catheter Cardiovasc Interv* 2006;**67**:250–3.
11. Lane RE, Ilsley CD, Wallis W, Dalby MC. Percutaneous coronary intervention of a circumflex chronic total occlusion using an epicardial collateral retrograde approach. *Catheter Cardiovasc Interv* 2006;**69**:842–4.
12. Rathore S, Katoh O, Matsuo H, et al. Retrograde percutaneous recanalization of chronic total occlusion of the coronary arteries: procedural outcomes and predictors of success in contemporary practice. *Circ Cardiovasc Interv* 2009;**2**:124–32.

13. Rathore S, Katoh O, Tuschikane E, Oida A, Suzuki T, Takase S. A novel modification of the retrograde approach for the recanalization of chronic total occlusion of the coronary arteries intravascular ultrasound-guided reverse controlled antegrade and retrograde tracking. *JACC Cardiovasc Interv* 2010;**3**:155−64.

14. Sianos G, Barlis P, Di Mario C, et al. European experience with the retrograde approach for the recanalisation of coronary artery chronic total occlusions. A report on behalf of the euroCTO club. *EuroIntervention* 2008;**4**:84−92.

15. Biondi-Zoccai GG, Bollati M, Moretti C, et al. Retrograde percutaneous recanalization of coronary chronic total occlusions: outcomes from 17 patients. *Int J Cardiol* 2008;**130**:118−20.

16. Galassi AR, Tomasello SD, Reifart N, et al. In-hospital outcomes of percutaneous coronary intervention in patients with chronic total occlusion: insights from the ERCTO (European Registry of Chronic Total Occlusion) registry. *EuroIntervention* 2011;**7**:472−9.

17. Thompson CA, Jayne JE, Robb JF, et al. Retrograde techniques and the impact of operator volume on percutaneous intervention for coronary chronic total occlusions an early U.S. experience. *JACC Cardiovasc Interv* 2009;**2**:834−42.

18. Karmpaliotis D, Michael TT, Brilakis ES, et al. Retrograde coronary chronic total occlusion revascularization: procedural and in-hospital outcomes from a multicenter registry in the United States. *JACC Cardiovasc Interv* 2012;**5**:1273−9.

19. Wu EB, Chan WW, Yu CM. Retrograde chronic total occlusion intervention: tips and tricks. *Catheter Cardiovasc Interv* 2008;**72**:806−14.

20. Fang HY, Wu CC, Wu CJ. Successful transradial antegrade coronary intervention of a rare right coronary artery high anterior downward takeoff anomalous chronic total occlusion by double-anchoring technique and retrograde guidance. *Int Heart J* 2009;**50**:531−8.

21. Nombela-Franco L, Werner GS. Retrograde recanalization of a chronic ostial occlusion of the left anterior descending artery: how to manage extreme takeoff angles. *J Invasive Cardiol* 2010;**22**:E7−12.

22. Kaneda H, Takahashi S, Saito S. Successful coronary intervention for chronic total occlusion in an anomalous right coronary artery using the retrograde approach via a collateral vessel. *J Invasive Cardiol* 2007;**19**:E1−4.

23. Marmagkiolis K, Brilakis ES, Hakeem A, Cilingiroglu M, Bilodeau L. Saphenous vein graft perforation during percutaneous coronary intervention: a case series. *J Invasive Cardiol* 2013;**25**:157−61.

24. Brilakis ES, Banerjee S, Lombardi WL. Retrograde recanalization of native coronary artery chronic occlusions via acutely occluded vein grafts. *Catheter Cardiovasc Interv* 2010;**75**:109−13.
25. Matsumi J, Adachi K, Saito S. A unique complication of the retrograde approach in angioplasty for chronic total occlusion of the coronary artery. *Catheter Cardiovasc Interv* 2008;**72**:371−8.
26. Aggarwal C, Varghese J, Uretsky BF. Left atrial inflow and outflow obstruction as a complication of retrograde approach for chronic total occlusion: report of a case and literature review of left atrial hematoma after percutaneous coronary intervention. *Catheter Cardiovasc Interv* 2012;**82**:770−5.
27. Werner GS, Ferrari M, Heinke S, et al. Angiographic assessment of collateral connections in comparison with invasively determined collateral function in chronic coronary occlusions. *Circulation* 2003;**107**:1972−7.
28. Brilakis ES, Badhey N, Banerjee S. "Bilateral knuckle" technique and Stingray re-entry system for retrograde chronic total occlusion intervention. *J Invasive Cardiol* 2011;**23**:E37−9.
29. Kawamura A, Jinzaki M, Kuribayashi S. Percutaneous revascularization of chronic total occlusion of left anterior descending artery using contralateral injection via isolated conus artery. *J Invasive Cardiol* 2009;**21**:E84−6.
30. Sianos G, Papafaklis MI. Septal wire entrapment during recanalisation of a chronic total occlusion with the retrograde approach. *Hellenic J Cardiol* 2011;**52**:79−83.
31. Lichtenwalter C, Banerjee S, Brilakis ES. Dual guide catheter technique for treating native coronary artery lesions through tortuous internal mammary grafts: separating equipment delivery from target lesion visualization. *J Invasive Cardiol* 2010;**22**:E78−81.
32. Saeed B, Banerjee S, Brilakis ES. Percutaneous coronary intervention in tortuous coronary arteries: associated complications and strategies to improve success. *J Interv Cardiol* 2008;**21**:504−11.
33. Kawasaki T, Koga H, Serikawa T. New bifurcation guidewire technique: a reversed guidewire technique for extremely angulated bifurcation—a case report. *Catheter Cardiovasc Interv* 2008;**71**:73−6.
34. Shirai S, Doijiri T, Iwabuchi M. Treatment for LMCA ostial stenosis using a bifurcation technique with a retrograde approach. *Catheter Cardiovasc Interv* 2010;**75**:748−52.
35. Routledge H, Lefevre T, Ohanessian A, Louvard Y, Dumas P, Morice MC. Use of a deflectable tip catheter to facilitate complex interventions beyond insertion of coronary bypass grafts: three case reports. *Catheter Cardiovasc Interv* 2007;**70**:862−6.

36. Iturbe JM, Abdel-Karim AR, Raja VN, Rangan BV, Banerjee S, Brilakis ES. Use of the venture wire control catheter for the treatment of coronary artery chronic total occlusions. *Catheter Cardiovasc Interv* 2010;**76**:936−41.

37. Saito S. Different strategies of retrograde approach in coronary angioplasty for chronic total occlusion. *Catheter Cardiovasc Interv* 2008;**71**:8−19.

38. Furuichi S, Satoh T. Intravascular ultrasound-guided retrograde wiring for chronic total occlusion. *Catheter Cardiovasc Interv* 2010;**75**:214−21.

39. Wu EB, Chan WW, Yu CM. Antegrade balloon transit of retrograde wire to bail out dissected left main during retrograde chronic total occlusion intervention—a variant of the reverse CART technique. *J Invasive Cardiol* 2009;**21**:e113−8.

40. Wu EB, Chan WW, Yu CM. The confluent balloon technique—two cases illustrating a novel method to achieve rapid wire crossing of chronic total occlusion during retrograde approach percutaneous coronary intervention. *J Invasive Cardiol* 2009;**21**:539−42.

41. Tsuchikane E, Katoh O, Kimura M, Nasu K, Kinoshita Y, Suzuki T. The first clinical experience with a novel catheter for collateral channel tracking in retrograde approach for chronic coronary total occlusions. *JACC Cardiovasc Interv* 2010;**3**:165−71.

42. Lee NH, Suh J, Seo HS. Double anchoring balloon technique for recanalization of coronary chronic total occlusion by retrograde approach. *Catheter Cardiovasc Interv* 2009;**73**:791−4.

43. Christ G, Glogar D. Successful recanalization of a chronic occluded left anterior descending coronary artery with a modification of the retrograde proximal true lumen puncture technique: the antegrade microcatheter probing technique. *Catheter Cardiovasc Interv* 2009;**73**:272−5.

44. Kim MH, Yu LH, Mitsudo K. A new retrograde wiring technique for chronic total occlusion. *Catheter Cardiovasc Interv* 2010;**75**:117−9.

45. Ge J, Zhang F. Retrograde recanalization of chronic total coronary artery occlusion using a novel "reverse wire trapping" technique. *Catheter Cardiovasc Interv* 2009;**74**:855−60.

46. Ng R, Hui PY, Beyer A, Ren X, Ochiai M. Successful retrograde recanalization of a left anterior descending artery chronic total occlusion through a previously placed left anterior descending-to-diagonal artery stent. *J Invasive Cardiol* 2010;**22**:E16−8.

47. Matsumi J, Saito S. Progress in the retrograde approach for chronic total coronary artery occlusion: a case with successful angioplasty

using CART and reverse-anchoring techniques 3 years after failed PCI via a retrograde approach. *Catheter Cardiovasc Interv* 2008;**71**:810−4.

48. Utunomiya M, Katoh O, Nakamura S. Percutaneous coronary intervention for a right coronary artery stent occlusion using retrograde delivery of a sirolimus-eluting stent via a septal perforator. *Catheter Cardiovasc Interv* 2009;**73**:475−80.

49. Bansal D, Uretsky BF. Treatment of chronic total occlusion by retrograde passage of stents through an epicardial collateral vessel. *Catheter Cardiovasc Interv* 2008;**72**:365−9.

50. Utsunomiya M, Kobayashi T, Nakamura S. Case of dislodged stent lost in septal channel during stent delivery in complex chronic total occlusion of right coronary artery. *J Invasive Cardiol* 2009;**21**:E229−33.

51. Michael TT, Papayannis AC, Banerjee S, Brilakis ES. Subintimal dissection/reentry strategies in coronary chronic total occlusion interventions. *Circ Cardiovasc Interv* 2012;**5**:729−38.

52. Ge JB, Zhang F, Ge L, Qian JY, Wang H. Wire trapping technique combined with retrograde approach for recanalization of chronic total occlusion. *Chin Med J (Engl)* 2008;**121**:1753−6.

53. Utsunomiya M, Mukohara N, Hirami R, Nakamura S. Percutaneous coronary intervention for chronic total occlusive lesion of a left anterior descending artery using the retrograde approach via a septal−septal channel. *Cardiovasc Revasc Med* 2010;**11**:34−40.

54. Otsuji S, Terasoma K, Takiuchi S. Retrograde recanalization of a left anterior descending chronic total occlusion via an ipsilateral intraseptal collateral. *J Invasive Cardiol* 2008;**20**:312−6.

55. Brilakis ES, Grantham JA, Banerjee S. "Ping-pong" guide catheter technique for retrograde intervention of a chronic total occlusion through an ipsilateral collateral. *Catheter Cardiovasc Interv* 2011;**78**:395−9.

7 Putting it all Together: The "Hybrid" Approach

The optimal approach to chronic total occlusion (CTO) percutaneous coronary intervention (PCI) continues to evolve. Although various CTO crossing techniques have been developed (antegrade wire escalation; antegrade dissection/re-entry; and retrograde, as described in Chapters 4–6), there are different schools of thought about the relative merits and priority of each of those approaches.

In January 2011, several high-volume CTO operators convened in a workshop that took place in Bellingham, Washington, and created a consensus algorithmic approach about how to optimally approach CTO crossing.[1] This approach has been named the "hybrid" approach to CTO PCI (Figure 7.1) and focuses on opening the occluded vessel, using all available techniques (antegrade, retrograde, true-to-true lumen crossing, or re-entry) tailored to the specific case in the most safe, effective, and efficient way.

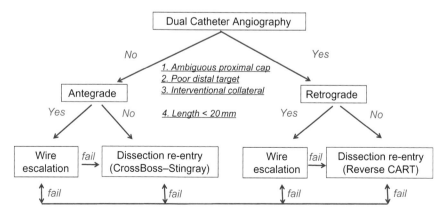

Figure 7.1 Overview of the "hybrid" CTO crossing algorithm.

Manual of Coronary Chronic Total Occlusion Interventions. DOI: http://dx.doi.org/10.1016/B978-0-12-420129-3.00007-6

The main principle behind the "hybrid" approach is that operators should master the entire skillsets of CTO PCI and be able to alternate between these techniques during the same CTO PCI procedure in order to recanalize the CTO. The goal has been to de-mystify the procedure by breaking down its various components and gaining in-depth understanding of the principles underlying each technique, and to make it reproducible and teachable, and thus available to the broader interventional community. The "hybrid" approach has been used in a large number of cases with high success rates and is also useful in learning CTO PCI in a stepwise fashion.

7.1 Description of the "Hybrid" Algorithm[2]

Step 1 Dual Injection

The first and arguably most important step of CTO PCI is to perform dual coronary injection, in nearly all cases, as described in detail in Section 3.2. Dual injection allows good visualization of both the proximal and the distal vessel, as well as the collateral circulation, allowing selection of the most suitable initial crossing technique. It also clarifies the location of the guidewire(s) during crossing attempts. Routine performance of dual injection is the simplest and most important step toward increasing the success rate and safety of CTO PCI.

Step 2 Assessment of CTO Characteristics

In-depth review of diagnostic angiographic images prior to PCI is critical. Most experienced CTO operators recommend against performing ad hoc CTO PCI, but rather performing CTO PCI only after a well-thought-out procedural plan is developed. Time spent studying the diagnostic film is an investment toward a successful CTO PCI procedure. Moreover, radiation and contrast can be reduced during PCI, since the anatomical information has already been obtained during diagnostic angiography. Sometimes, however, dual injection images may not be performed until the time of PCI.

Four angiographic parameters are assessed: (a) the morphology of the proximal cap (clear-cut or ambiguous); (b) the length of the occlusion; (c) the vessel size and presence of bifurcations beyond the distal cap (i.e., "landing zone"); and (d) the location and suitability of collateral channels for retrograde access (Figure 7.2):[1]

1. **Proximal cap location and morphology.** This characteristic refers to the ability to unambiguously localize the entry point to the CTO lesion by angiography or intravascular ultrasonography (Figure 4.11) and to understand the course of the vessel in the CTO segment.

    For example, a favorable proximal cap is one that is tapered, as opposed to being blunt, and has no bridging collaterals or major side branches that would make engagement of the CTO segment difficult using traditional wire escalation techniques. A particularly challenging anatomic subset is that of blunt ostial occlusions, which often requires use of the retrograde approach.

2. **Lesion length.** Lesions are dichotomized into those that are <20 and ≥ 20 mm long.[3] As noted above, in most cases this characteristic can only be accurately assessed by using dual injections.

    In CTOs in which antegrade crossing is attempted, short CTOs (<20 mm) are usually best approached with antegrade wiring, whereas in long (≥ 20 mm) CTOs, upfront use of a subintimal dissection/re-entry technique is preferred, because there is high probability that wire-based crossing attempts will result in subintimal wire entry. A lesion length of <20 mm has been identified as a predictor of rapid CTO crossing in J-CTO (Multicenter CTO Registry in Japan— Figure 7.3).[3] With the wide adoption of dual injection, it has become evident that the length of the occlusion is frequently shorter than estimated by single injections.

3. **Target coronary vessel beyond the distal cap.** This refers to the size of the lumen, presence of significant side branches, vessel disease at

Anatomy Dictates Strategy

Four questions

1. Clear or ambiguous proximal cap

2. Lesion length ($<$ or $\geq$ 20 mm)

3. Quality of the distal target

4. "Interventional" collaterals

Figure 7.2 Key anatomic characteristics for selecting a CTO crossing strategy.

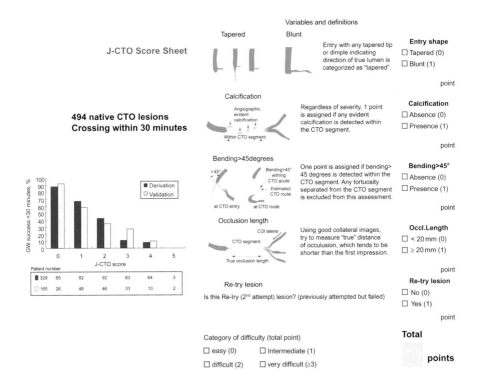

Figure 7.3 Calculation of the J-CTO score to determine the difficulty of CTO crossing.
Source: Reproduced with permission from Ref. 3.

the reconstitution point, and ability to adequately angiographically visualize this segment.

4. **Size and suitability of collateral circulation** for retrograde techniques. Optimal collateral vessels for retrograde CTO PCI:

   a. Are sourced from a healthy (or repaired) donor vessel.
   b. Can be easily accessed with wires and microcatheters.
   c. Have minimal tortuosity.
   d. Are not the only source of flow to the CTO segment (which places the patient at risk for intraprocedural ischemia during crossing of the collateral).
   e. Enter the CTO vessel well beyond the distal cap.

   More favorable collateral circulation characteristics lower the barriers to utilizing retrograde techniques as an initial strategy or as an early crossover strategy.

What constitutes an "interventional" collateral (i.e., a collateral that can be wired during a retrograde approach) varies depending upon the experience and skills of the operator. In-depth understanding of the collateral circulation is also of paramount importance during antegrade crossing attempts, since dissection re-entry techniques and the formation of subintimal hematomas may compromise ipsilateral or bridging collaterals, leading to poor visualization of the distal vessel at the re-entry zone and occasionally ischemia (Chapter 6). Degenerated or even occluded bypass grafts anastomosed to the target vessel can also be used as retrograde conduits to facilitate PCI.[4,5]

Assessment and utilization of the above four angiographic characteristics is highly dependent on operator experience and skillset and is thus constantly evolving.

Step 3 Antegrade Wiring (Chapter 4)

Antegrade wire escalation refers to the use of guidewires of increasing stiffness to cross a CTO. In the past, a "gradual" escalation was performed: starting with a workhorse guidewire and then increasing to a Miracle 3, 6, 9, and eventually Confianza Pro 12 guidewire. Currently, however, a more rapid escalation is favored from a tapered-tip polymer-jacketed guidewire (Fielder XT) to either a stiff polymer-jacketed wire (Pilot 200) when the course of the CTO is uncertain or a stiff, tapered tip guidewire (Confianza Pro 12) in cases where the course of the CTO is well understood. Streamlined use of a relatively small array of guidewires can simplify clinical decisions and inventory management and also leads to in-depth understanding of the properties of the different wires.

Step 4 Antegrade Dissection and Re-Entry (Chapter 5)

For long lesions approached in the antegrade direction, upfront use of a dissection/re-entry strategy is recommended (Figure 7.4). Dissection can be achieved either by advancing a "knuckle" formed at the tip of a polymer-jacketed guidewire (such as the Fielder XT or the Pilot 200) or by using the CrossBoss catheter. Antegrade dissection minimizes the risk for perforation (by the blunt guidewire loop or by the CrossBoss catheter tip)

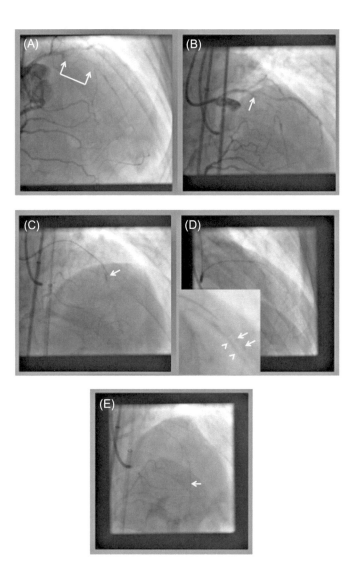

Figure 7.4 Example of antegrade/dissection re-entry. Coronary angiography demonstrating a CTO of the mid left anterior descending artery (arrows, A). Angiographic characteristics included well-visualized proximal cap, good distal target, and lesion length >20 mm (H). A CrossBoss catheter was advanced to the proximal cap (arrow, B). Using the fast-spin technique, the catheter crossed the occlusion subintimally into the mid left anterior descending artery (arrow, C). The CrossBoss catheter was exchanged for a Stingray balloon (arrows, D), located adjacent to the true lumen (arrowheads, D). A Stingray guidewire (arrow, E) successfully crossed into the distal true lumen. Angiography after predilation showed expected dissection at the area of subintimal crossing (arrows, F). After implantation of multiple drug-eluting stents an excellent angiographic result was achieved (G).
Source: Reproduced with permission from Ref. 1.

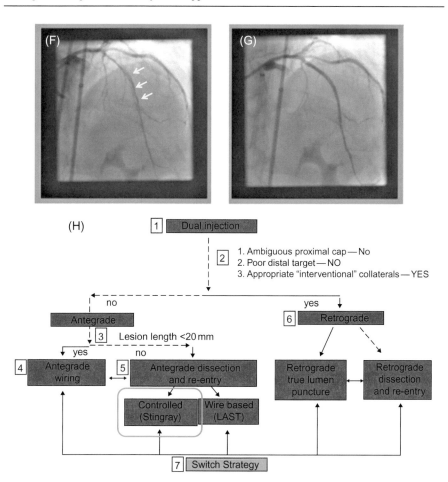

Figure 7.4 (Continued)

and allows for rapid crossing of long occlusion segments. Re-entry can be achieved using a stiff polymer-jacketed or tapered-tip guidewire with a sharp distal bend, or more consistently by using the Stingray system, as described in Chapter 5, Step 4.

Once a particular strategy is selected based on the "hybrid" algorithm (e.g., Stingray-based re-entry), the operator should resist the temptation of "regressing" into more conventional techniques, such as attempts to re-enter using different wires, as such attempts may expand the subintimal space and hinder re-entry, ultimately leading to a failed procedure.

Step 5 Retrograde (Chapter 6)

The retrograde approach is a major component of a contemporary CTO PCI program. The retrograde approach can be used either upfront (primary retrograde, Figure 7.5) or after a failed antegrade crossing attempt, and it enables high procedural success rates.[6−8] Factors that favor a primary retrograde approach include an ambiguous proximal cap, poor distal target, good interventional collaterals, and also heavy calcification and chronic kidney disease (as the retrograde approach has lower contrast requirements). Retrograde wire crossing can occur by advancing the retrograde guidewire into the proximal true lumen (retrograde true lumen puncture, conceptually similar to antegrade wire escalation), by antegrade wiring toward a retrograde-placed guidewire into the distal true lumen ("just marker" technique), or by using one of the dissection/re-entry techniques, such as controlled antegrade and retrograde tracking (CART), or, more commonly, the reverse CART technique, as described in Chapter 6.

Step 6 Change

Alternating between different CTO PCI techniques is at the heart of the "hybrid" algorithm (Figure 7.6). When one approach fails, something different should be attempted. For example, if antegrade wire crossing fails, then antegrade dissection/re-entry should be tried, and if this fails too, retrograde crossing should be attempted (if, of course, appropriate collaterals exist).

Every CTO is different and as a result may require different strategies for success. Excessive persistence in the face of minimal progress increases the chances for procedural failure due to utilization of limited resources (radiation, contrast, time). However, the operator should not change too early, but instead invest enough effort in the utilized strategy to maximize its chance for success. What constitutes an "adequate effort" varies from lesion to lesion and operator to operator and is best determined with increased CTO PCI experience. Generally, no more than 5−10 min should be spent in a stagnant mode without minor (such as re-shaping the wire tip or changing to a wire with significantly different properties), or major (such as switching from an antegrade to a retrograde approach) technique adjustments being made. Efficient change of strategy can result in shorter procedure time and lower patient and staff radiation exposure, and contrast utilization. The "hybrid" approach message is: Do

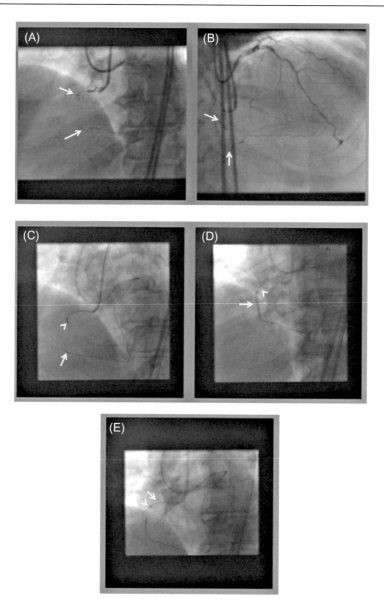

Figure 7.5 Primary retrograde percutaneous coronary intervention to a right coronary artery CTO. Dual coronary angiography demonstrating a CTO of the proximal right coronary artery (arrows, A and B) with distal filling via collaterals from the left anterior descending artery. The angiographic characterization was poorly identified proximal cap, long lesion, diffusely diseased distal target, and good interventional collaterals (H).

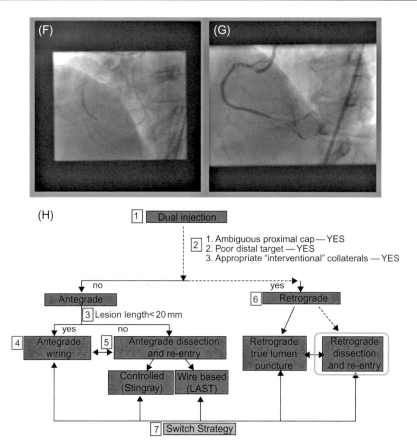

Figure 7.5 (Continued)

◄ A Corsair microcatheter (arrow, C) was advanced retrograde via a septal collateral over a soft, polymer-jacketed, non-tapered guidewire, to the distal right coronary artery. A second Corsair microcatheter (arrowhead, C) was advanced antegrade to the mid right coronary artery. After antegrade insertion of a Guideliner catheter (arrowhead, D), a 2.5 × 20 mm balloon was inflated over the antegrade guidewire in the mid right coronary artery (arrow, D) and reverse controlled antegrade and retrograde tracking and dissection (reverse CART) was performed, followed by successful advancement of a retrograde Pilot 200 guidewire (E) into the antegrade Guideliner. A ViperWire Advance 335-cm guidewire was externalized followed by predilation of the right coronary artery (F) and restoration of antegrade flow after implantation of multiple drug-eluting stents (G). *Source*: Reproduced with permission from Ref. 1.

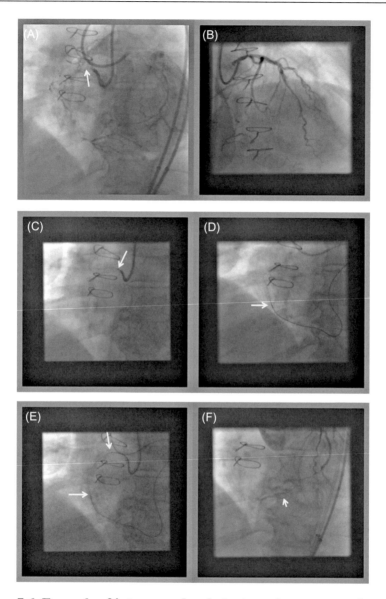

Figure 7.6 Example of intraprocedural strategy changes: complex antegrade and retrograde intervention of a right coronary artery CTO. Bilateral coronary angiography demonstrating a proximal right coronary artery CTO due to in-stent restenosis (arrow, A). The right posterior descending artery filled by septal collaterals from the left anterior descending artery (B). Angiographic characteristics included well-defined proximal cap, good distal target, long lesion length, and appropriate retrograde "interventional collaterals." Antegrade crossing attempts using a CrossBoss catheter (arrow, C) and antegrade wire escalation failed. A Corsair microcatheter (arrow, D) was advanced retrograde via a septal

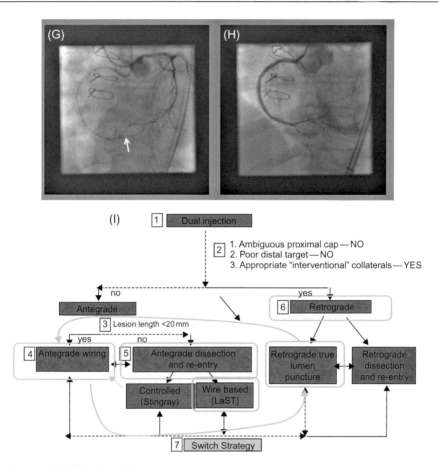

Figure 7.6 (Continued)

collateral to the mid right coronary artery over a non-tapered polymer-jacketed guidewire but attempts to cross the occlusion retrograde failed (E). Repeat antegrade crossing attempts with a moderately stiff, non-tapered polymer-jacketed wire (Pilot 200 wire) using limited antegrade subintimal tracking (LAST) technique were successful in subintimal advancement of the wire (arrow, F). After a Guideliner catheter (arrowhead, G) was advanced into the proximal right coronary artery, a Confianza Pro 12 wire (arrow, G) successfully crossed the occlusion into the distal true lumen. After implantation of multiple drug-eluting stents an excellent angiographic result was achieved (H).

This case highlights the importance of multiple modifications in the procedural plan (I), and "switching" strategies to be adaptive during CTO PCI interventions.

Source: Reproduced with permission from Ref. 1.

not let the case stall! The "hybrid" approach requires a high level of familiarity and comfort with all crossing strategies, so that there are no impe-
diments to making a change.

7.2   Impact of the "Hybrid" Approach

The "hybrid" approach algorithm has had a major impact on the dis-
semination and application of CTO PCI techniques in recent years,
by a wider population of interventional cardiologists, in different
practice settings (from small private practice groups, to academic
institutions, to non-academic tertiary centers). It allowed for the first
time an approach to CTO PCI in a simple (but not simplistic), systematic, reproducible, and teachable way.

An initial single operator experience with "hybrid" CTO PCI is
demonstrated in Figure 7.7.[9] A change in the CTO crossing strategy
was required in approximately half the cases.

A "hybrid registry" of 144 cases performed between January 2011
and October 2012 was presented at the 2012 CTO Summit. All cases
had been previously recorded during "hybrid" workshops at five centers in the United States. The data was abstracted independently by
nonparticipants. Overall procedural success was 94%, with efficient
use of resources (average procedure time was 85 min and average
contrast utilization was 238 mL). The average J-CTO score was 2.3,
with over 46% of lesions having a J-CTO score >3, demonstrating a
high degree of lesion complexity. Despite this, there was no decre-
ment in success rates (92.5%) in the most complex lesion subset (J-
CTO >3) using a variety of strategies (Figure 7.8). This appeared to
be at least in part due to the "change" aspect of the hybrid algorithm,
with a considerable increase in the use of secondary and tertiary strategies for successful results in the more complex lesions.

Full application of the CTO "hybrid" algorithm requires long-term
commitment, ongoing training, and experience with all types of CTO
PCI techniques, and hence may not be fully applicable to all operators
at different stages of their learning curve. It does provide, however, a
framework of effective communication between operators that can
facilitate acquiring and building a comprehensive CTO PCI skillset.

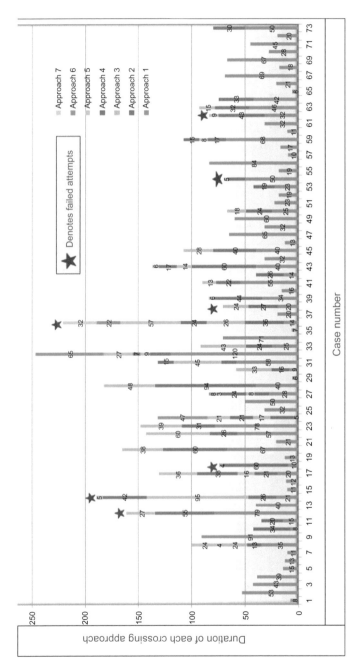

Figure 7.7 Application of the "hybrid" approach in a single operator registry. The number of CTO crossing approach changes among 73 consecutive CTO PCI cases was recorded. Overall success rate was 90.4% and 32 of 73 patients (44%) required 3.6 ± 1.4 approach changes. The final successful crossing technique was antegrade wire escalation in 50%, antegrade dissection/re-entry in 24.2%, and retrograde in 25.8%. *Source:* Reproduced with permission from Ref. 9.

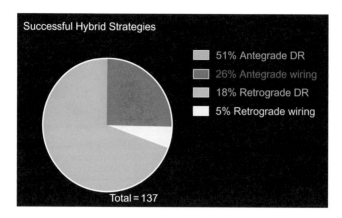

Figure 7.8 Successful crossing strategies among 137 successful cases in a North American "hybrid registry."
Source: Courtesy of Dr. David Daniels.

References

1. Brilakis ES, Grantham JA, Rinfret S, et al. A percutaneous treatment algorithm for crossing coronary chronic total occlusions. *JACC Cardiovasc Interv* 2012;**5**:367–79.
2. Brilakis ES. The "hybrid" approach: the key to CTO crosing success. *Cardiol Today's Interv* 2012. (November/December).
3. Morino Y, Abe M, Morimoto T, et al. Predicting successful guidewire crossing through chronic total occlusion of native coronary lesions within 30 minutes: the J-CTO (Multicenter CTO Registry in Japan) score as a difficulty grading and time assessment tool. *JACC Cardiovasc Interv* 2011;**4**:213–21.
4. Kahn JK, Hartzler GO. Retrograde coronary angioplasty of isolated arterial segments through saphenous vein bypass grafts. *Cathet Cardiovasc Diagn* 1990;**20**:88–93.
5. Brilakis ES, Banerjee S, Lombardi WL. Retrograde recanalization of native coronary artery chronic occlusions via acutely occluded vein grafts. *Catheter Cardiovasc Interv* 2010;**75**:109–13.
6. Rathore S, Katoh O, Matsuo H, et al. Retrograde percutaneous recanalization of chronic total occlusion of the coronary arteries: procedural outcomes and predictors of success in contemporary practice. *Circ Cardiovasc Interv* 2009;**2**:124–32.
7. Karmpaliotis D, Michael TT, Brilakis ES, et al. Retrograde coronary chronic total occlusion revascularization: procedural and in-hospital

outcomes from a multicenter registry in the United States. *JACC Cardiovasc Interv* 2012;**5**:1273−9.

8. Tsuchikane E, Yamane M, Mutoh M, et al. Japanese multicenter registry evaluating the retrograde approach for chronic coronary total occlusion. *Catheter Cardiovasc Interv* 2013;**82**:E654−61.

9. Michael TT, Mogabgab O, Fuh E, et al. Application of the "Hybrid Approach" To Chronic Total Occlusion Interventions: a Detailed Procedural Analysis. *J Interv Cardiol* 2013 [published online before print].

8 "Balloon Uncrossable" CTOs

Goal: Cross the chronic total occlusion (CTO) with a balloon after successful guidewire crossing.

The main reason for failure of CTO interventions is inability to cross the occlusion with a guidewire. However, in few cases a balloon cannot cross the lesion after successful guidewire crossing and confirmation of guidewire placement into the distal true lumen. Such lesions are called "balloon uncrossable" CTOs. Figure 8.1 outlines a step-by-step algorithm for approaching such lesions.

Step 1 Advancing/Inflating a Small Balloon
How?

a. Use single marker, rapid exchange balloons with low-crossing profile (1.20, 1.25, or 1.5 mm in diameter) and long length (20−30 mm). The balloon profile is highest at the marker segment; hence, longer balloons may allow deeper lesion penetration before the balloon marker reaches the proximal cap of the CTO.

b. If the balloon stops advancing, it can be inflated while maintaining forward pressure. This may dilate the proximal cap and allow lesion crossing, sometimes even with the same balloon.

c. If the balloon fails to advance after inflation, one can try with a new small balloon (since balloons do not return to their original profile after inflation), or one manufactured by another company, as different crossing profile and tip confirmation may assist in crossing. Rapid exchange balloon catheters allow more pushability into the stenosis.

d. Alternatively, one can attempt crossing with a larger 2.5−3.0-mm diameter rapid exchange balloon. Sometimes inflation with a larger diameter balloon just proximal to the CTO lesion will disrupt the architecture of the proximal CTO cap enough to allow subsequent passage of a small profile balloon.

Manual of Coronary Chronic Total Occlusion Interventions. DOI: http://dx.doi.org/10.1016/B978-0-12-420129-3.00008-8

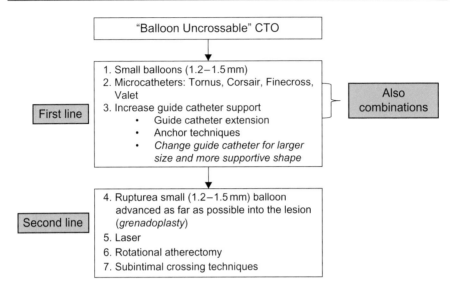

Figure 8.1 Algorithm for crossing a "balloon uncrossable" CTO.

What can go wrong?

— Guide catheter and guidewire position can be lost during attempts to advance the balloon. Watch carefully the guide catheter position and stop advancing if the guide catheter starts backing out of the coronary ostium or if the distal wire position is being compromised.
— Injury of the distal target vessel can occur (dissection or perforation) in case of significant distal guidewire movement ("see-saw" action of wire with forward push of balloon and retraction of force), especially when stiff (such as Confianza Pro 12) or polymer-jacketed (such as the Pilot 200) guidewires are used.

Step 2 Advancing a Microcatheter
How?

a. The Tornus catheter (Section 2.7.1) was designed for advancing through calcified and difficult to penetrate lesions and should be advanced using counterclockwise rotation.[1]
b. The Corsair catheter (Section 2.3.2) can be advanced by rotating in either direction (in contrast to the Tornus catheter).

c. Other microcatheters can also be used, such as the Finecross (Section 2.3.3) or the Valet (Section 2.3.4) catheter. Rotation can be performed in either direction, similar to the Corsair.

d. If successful advancement of a specialty microcatheter is achieved, a balloon can often cross the lesion as well. Alternatively, the guidewire could be exchanged for a rotational atherectomy wire, if the latter is planned as the next debulking step.

What can go wrong?

— Guide catheter and guidewire position may be lost with aggressive pushing of the microcatheters.
— Distal vessel injury can occur from uncontrolled guidewire movement during microcatheter advancement attempts.
— The Tornus catheter can get damaged if over-torqued, leading to catheter entrapment or shaft breakage. Counterclockwise rotation should not exceed 10 turns before allowing the catheter to "unwind."
— Rarely excessive manipulation of the Corsair can disrupt the device and/or the guidewire and lock both devices together requiring withdrawal of both. The Fielder XT guidewire may allow rewiring through the original channel and the crossing attempts to restart.

Step 3 Increasing Guide Catheter Support

How?

Guide catheter support can be enhanced by using a side-branch anchor technique,[2] or a guide catheter extension,[3] as described in detail in Section 3.6:

a. Side-branch anchor technique. A workhorse guidewire is advanced into a side branch (usually a conus or acute marginal branch for the right coronary artery (RCA) or a diagonal for the left anterior descending artery, LAD), followed by a small balloon (usually 1.5—2.0 mm in diameter depending on the side-branch vessel size) (Figure 8.2). The balloon is inflated usually at 6—8 atm "anchoring" the guide into the vessel and enhancing advancement of balloons or microcatheters.

b. Guide catheter extension. A Guideliner, Guidezilla, or Heartrail (the Heartrail is not currently available in the United States) catheter is advanced into the vessel, enhancing guide catheter support and the pushability of balloons/microcatheters. Use of a guide catheter extension can also decrease the amount of contrast injected and provide improved visualization via subselective coronary artery engagement.

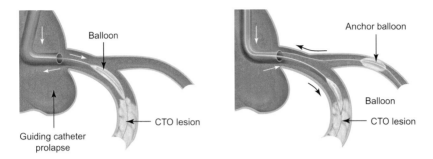

Figure 8.2 Example of side-branch anchor to facilitate delivery of a balloon across a CTO.

In a recent randomized trial, use of a 5-in-6 guide catheter extension was more effective and efficient in facilitating the success of transradial PCI for complex coronary lesions, compared to buddy-wire or balloon-anchoring approach.[4]

What can go wrong?

— Guidewire and guide catheter position loss or distal vessel injury.
— Side-branch anchor can cause injury or dissection of the side branch, but this is infrequent and usually does not have adverse consequences.
— Perforation of the side branch may rarely occur. Oversizing of the anchor balloon should be avoided to minimize the risk for both side-branch perforation and dissection.
— Guide catheter extensions can cause ostial or mid target vessel dissection.[3]

Step 4 Grenadoplasty (Intentional Balloon Rupture; also Called "Balloon-Assisted Microdissection"—BAM)

How?

A small (usually 1.20—1.50 mm) balloon is advanced as far as possible into the lesion and inflated at high pressure until it ruptures. The balloon rupture can modify the plaque resulting in successful penetration with another balloon.

What can go wrong?

— Proximal vessel dissection and perforation.
— Difficulty removing the ruptured balloon.

Step 5 Laser
How?

a. The 0.9-mm Excimer laser coronary atherectomy (ELCA) laser should be used at maximum repetition and fluence levels (repetition rate 80 Hz and fluence of 80 mJ/mm^2).[5] The laser may modify the proximal cap and facilitate balloon entry into the lesion.[6] Flushing with saline should be performed during passes of the laser catheter.[7]

b. **Variation of the above technique** (advanced technique that may carry risk for vessel injury and/or perforation): Perform laser using the over-the-wire laser catheter while injecting a mixture of 30% contrast/70% saline via the over-the-wire catheter side port using a Y-connector and an inflating device inflated up to 20 atm. Laser activation in contrast causes vaporization of the plaque by the accoustomechanical effect of the rapidly exploding bubbles.

What can go wrong?

— Vessel perforation, which is why the smallest caliber laser catheter is used and the true lumen distal location of the crossing guidewire should be first confirmed before attempting to advance the laser catheter.

— Avoid laser if CTO crossing was achieved using dissection/re-entry to minimize the risk for perforation.

Step 6 Rotational Atherectomy
How?

— Rotational atherectomy can greatly facilitate lesion crossing with a balloon. However, rotational atherectomy requires wire exchange for a 0.009-in. dedicated guidewire, which may not always be feasible through the CTO.[8]

— If no other maneuver is successful in crossing the CTO, one could consider burying an over-the-wire microcatheter as far into the CTO lesion as possible, then pulling the CTO wire and attempting to re-wire the CTO with a rotational atherectomy guidewire. If rewiring is successful, then rotational atherectomy can be performed.

— Rotational atherectomy may be safer than laser, as the burr will differentially cut calcific tissue but will not cut through elastic adventitia.

What can go wrong?

— Loss of guidewire position across the CTO (guidewire has to be removed and replaced with a rotational atherectomy guidewire) that may fail to recross the lesion.
— Vessel perforation, which is why a small diameter burr (1.25—1.50 mm) is usually used.
— Burr entrapment upon forceful forward advancement. The burr should be advanced in a repetitive and gentle manner avoiding forceful "wedging" into the occlusion. Prevention and management of this complication is discussed in Chapter 12.

Step 7 Subintimal Crossing Techniques

How?

a. A second guidewire is advanced subintimally distal to the CTO (or the CrossBoss catheter is used to achieve subintimal position and exchanged for the guidewire), as explained in Chapter 5 (Figure 8.3A—C). If the subintimal guidewire re-enters into the distal true lumen (Figure 8.3C), it can be used for balloon angioplasty and stenting instead of the original wire. A balloon is advanced over the subintimal guidewire next to the CTO and inflated (usually at 8—10 atm), "crushing" the CTO plaque from the outside (Figure 8.3D1). This can modify the plaque enough to allow passage of a balloon over the guidewire that has entered the distal true lumen.
b. In a variation of this technique entitled "subintimal distal anchor," a second guidewire is advanced subintimally distal to the CTO. A balloon is advanced over the subintimal guidewire distal to the CTO. The balloon is inflated distally, "anchoring" the true lumen guidewire, and enabling antegrade delivery of a balloon over the true lumen guidewire (Figure 8.3D2).

What can go wrong?

— The subintimal techniques require subintimal wire crossing, which may not always be feasible (e.g., the guidewire may track side branches).
— Positioning of the subintimal guidewire within the vessel "architecture" needs to be confirmed to prevent inadvertent perforation, for example, if the guidewire enters side branches.
— Subintimal crossing can cause subintimal hematoma that may compress the distal true lumen.

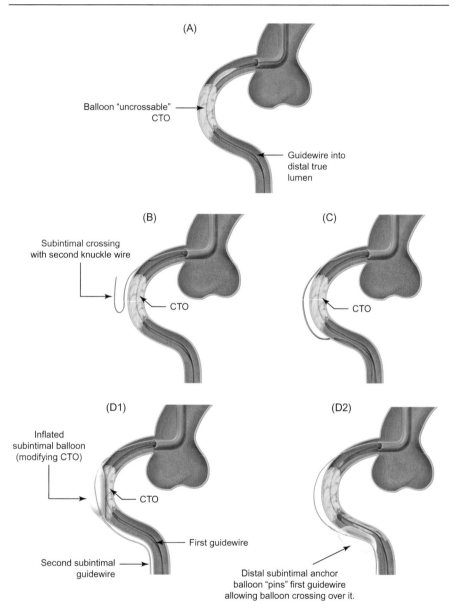

Figure 8.3 Illustration of subintimal crossing techniques for crossing a "balloon uncrossable" CTO. If a balloon cannot cross the CTO after successful guidewire crossing (A), a second guidewire is used to subintimally cross the CTO (B) and possibly re-enter into the distal true lumen (C). Alternatively if the subintimal wire does cannot enter into the distal true lumen, a balloon can be inflated over the subintimal guidewire next to the CTO to "crush" and modify it (D1), or distal to the CTO to "anchor" the true lumen guidewire and allow balloon crossing over the true lumen guidewire (D2).

8.1 Simultaneous Use of Strategies

Simultaneous application of lesion modification strategies and techniques that increase guide catheter support can enhance the likelihood of successful crossing: for example, the "Anchor-Tornus,"[9] "Proxis-Tornus,"[10] and "Anchor-Laser" (Figure 8.4)[5] techniques have been described for crossing "balloon uncrossable" lesions. In addition to simultaneous, sequential application of various techniques is used until a final successful outcome (Figure 8.5).[11] One must be creative when using the above strategies in various combinations to achieve the desired goal. The process can be difficult but also very rewarding.

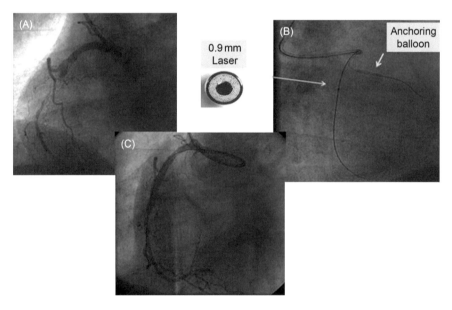

Figure 8.4 Example of combined use of side-branch anchoring and laser to cross a "balloon uncrossable" CTO. An RCA CTO (A) was successfully crossed with a guidewire but no balloon would cross the lesion. A laser catheter could not be delivered but did cross with use of a side-branch anchor balloon (B) enabling an excellent final angiographic result after stenting (C).
Source: Reproduced with permission from Ref. 5.

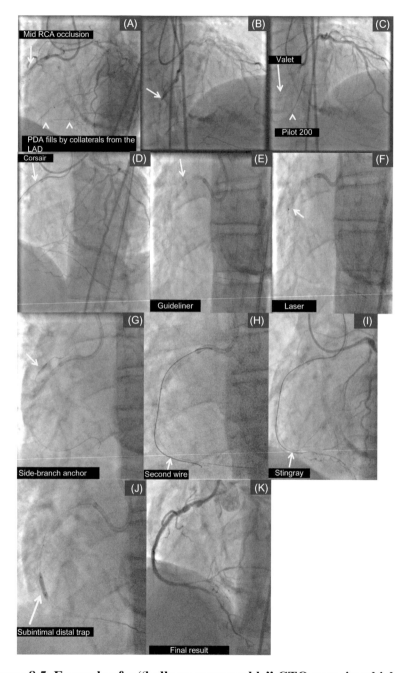

Figure 8.5 Example of a "balloon uncrossable" CTO case, in which multiple strategies were used as part of the algorithm proposed in Figure 8.1. Coronary angiography using dual injection demonstrating a

References

1. Fang HY, Lee CH, Fang CY, et al. Application of penetration device (Tornus) for percutaneous coronary intervention in balloon uncrossable chronic total occlusion-procedure outcomes, complications, and predictors of device success. *Catheter Cardiovasc Interv* 2011;**78**:356−62.
2. Di Mario C, Ramasami N. Techniques to enhance guide catheter support. *Catheter Cardiovasc Interv* 2008;**72**:505−12.
3. Luna M, Papayannis A, Holper EM, Banerjee S, Brilakis ES. Transfemoral use of the GuideLiner catheter in complex coronary and bypass graft interventions. *Catheter Cardiovasc Interv* 2012;**80**:437−46.
4. Zhang Q, Zhang RY, Kirtane AJ, et al. The utility of a 5-in-6 double catheter technique in treating complex coronary lesions via transradial approach: the DOCA-TRI study. *EuroIntervention* 2012;**8**:848−54.
5. Ben-Dor I, Maluenda G, Pichard AD, et al. The use of excimer laser for complex coronary artery lesions. *Cardiovasc Revasc Med* 2011;**12**(69): e1−8.
6. Niccoli G, Giubilato S, Conte M, et al. Laser for complex coronary lesions: impact of excimer lasers and technical advancements. *Int J Cardiol* 2011;**146**:296−9.
7. Shen ZJ, Garcia-Garcia HM, Schultz C, van der Ent M, Serruys PW. Crossing of a calcified "balloon uncrossable" coronary chronic total occlusion facilitated by a laser catheter: a case report and review recent four years' experience at the Thoraxcenter. *Int J Cardiol* 2010; **145**:251−4.

◄ CTO of the mid RCA (arrow, A). The posterior descending artery (PDA, arrowheads, A) filled via collaterals from the LAD. Dual injection coronary angiography showing a long mid RCA occlusion (arrow, B). The RCA CTO was successfully crossed using a Pilot 200 guidewire (arrowhead, C) over a Valet microcatheter (arrow, C). A Corsair catheter (arrow, D) failed to cross the lesion, in spite of use of a Guideliner (arrow, E) and 0.9-mm laser catheter (arrow, F). Crossing of the CTO with a balloon failed after use of a side-branch anchor balloon (arrow, G). The CTO was crossed subintimally with a second guidewire that was knuckled to the distal RCA (H), but re-entry attempts using the Stingray balloon and guidewire failed (arrow, I). A 3.0-mm balloon was inflated over the subintimal guidewire in the distal RCA (arrow, J) that "anchored" the true lumen guidewire allowing advancement of a 1.5-mm balloon through the CTO, enabling lesion dilation. After stenting an excellent final result was achieved (K). *Source*: Reproduced with permission from HMP Communications.[11]

8. Pagnotta P, Briguori C, Mango R, et al. Rotational atherectomy in resistant chronic total occlusions. *Catheter Cardiovasc Interv* 2010;**76**:366−71.
9. Kirtane AJ, Stone GW. The Anchor-Tornus technique: a novel approach to "uncrossable" chronic total occlusions. *Catheter Cardiovasc Interv* 2007;**70**:554−7.
10. Brilakis ES, Banerjee S. The "Proxis-Tornus" technique for a difficult-to-cross calcified saphenous vein graft lesion. *J Invasive Cardiol* 2008;**20**:E258−61.
11. Michael TT, Banerjee S, Brilakis ES. Subintimal distal anchor technique for "balloon-uncrossable" chronic total occlusions. *J Invasive Cardiol* 2013;**25**:552−4.

9 "Balloon Undilatable" CTOs

Goal: Dilate the lesion that does not expand in spite of multiple balloon inflations.

Prevention: "Balloon undilatable" lesions are more frequent in chronic total occlusions (CTOs) compared to non-CTO lesions. It is important to avoid implanting a stent in a "balloon undilatable" lesion. Adequate predilation with a balloon sized according to the vessel reference diameter is critical before stenting a CTO lesion to ensure proper stent expansion, especially when the lesion is severely calcified. If the lesion is resistant, additional predilation and/or plaque debulking strategies should be used before a stent is deployed.

Treatment: Figure 9.1 outlines an algorithm for approaching "balloon undilatable" CTOs.

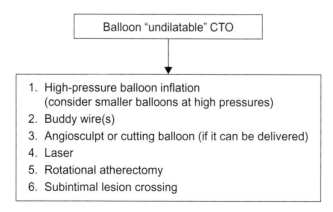

Figure 9.1 Proposed algorithm for dilating a "balloon undilatable" CTO.

Manual of Coronary Chronic Total Occlusion Interventions. DOI: http://dx.doi.org/10.1016/B978-0-12-420129-3.00009-X

Step 1 High-Pressure Balloon Inflation
How?

a. Using non-compliant balloons inflated at high pressures (often up to 30 atm).[1] Specialized non-compliant balloons have been developed to deliver very high (>40 atm) pressures (Schwager OPN balloon, SIS Medical, Switzerland) but are not currently available in the United States.[1] It is important to be familiar with the rated burst pressure and percentage diameter growth of the available non-compliant balloons.
b. Performing prolonged inflations (30−60 s).
c. Using slightly undersized balloons (usually by 0.5 mm).
d. Avoiding balloon injury of non-stented vessel segments. All ballooned segments should subsequently be covered with stent(s) to minimize the risk for restenosis.

What can go wrong?

a. Vessel perforation: Best avoided by conservative balloon sizing (in nearly all cases 1:1 or lower balloon to vessel ratio should be used).
b. Balloon rupture leading to vessel dissection and/or perforation.

Step 2 Buddy Wire(s)
How?

• Advancing one[2−4] or more[5] buddy wires through the undilatable CTO, followed by high-pressure balloon inflation: The wires can modify the balloon forces exerted on the vessel wall, leading to vessel modification and expansion (this is a "poor man's" version of cutting balloon or Angiosculpt use).

What can go wrong?

• Vessel injury from advancement of the buddy wire(s): using soft work-horse guidewires and careful wiring technique is advised. The buddy wire may inadvertently enter the subintimal space during advancement. Subintimal advancement could be prevented by using the Twin Pass catheter for buddy wire delivery.

Step 3 Angiosculpt or Cutting Balloon
How?

• Similar to the "buddy wire" technique, the vessel wall is modified by application of focused pressure through the blades of the cutting balloon[6] or nitinol wire of the Angiosculpt balloon (described in Section 2.7.3).

What can go wrong?

a. Loss of guidewire and guide catheter position, as the Angiosculpt or cutting balloon may not deliver easily through the "balloon undilatable" lesion: Use of enhanced guide catheter support techniques (such as anchor techniques and guide catheter extensions) may be needed to deliver the Angiosculpt or cutting balloon through the lesion.
b. Vessel rupture or perforation.
c. Balloon entrapment (especially if the balloon ruptures). Excessive inflation forces or balloon rupture within the lesion may make equipment withdrawal challenging.[7] The cutting balloon should be inflated slowly and >14 atm inflation pressures should be avoided.

Step 4 Laser

Use of laser can be effective in dilating "balloon undilatable" lesions[8,9] but does carry risk for perforation and dissection, especially if crossing was achieved using dissection/re-entry.[10] An aggressive variant of laser (laser angioplasty while flushing with contrast) can be more effective but also carries higher risk, as discussed in Step 4 of Chapter 8.[8,11] Laser may not be as effective in lesions with circumferential calcium, in which rotational atherectomy provides better results.

Step 5 Rotational Atherectomy

Rotational atherectomy has been successfully used to expand a "balloon undilatable" lesion, as discussed in Step 6 in Chapter 8.

Step 6 Subintimal Lesion Crossing

This may also allow expansion of the lesion, as discussed in Step 7 in Chapter 8.

9.1   Special Case Scenario: Stented "Balloon Undilatable" Lesions

Discovering that a lesion is "balloon undilatable" *after* stenting poses significant challenges, because stent underexpansion can predispose to stent thrombosis and restenosis (Figure 9.2). All steps described above can be used to expand the lesion and the deployed stent but

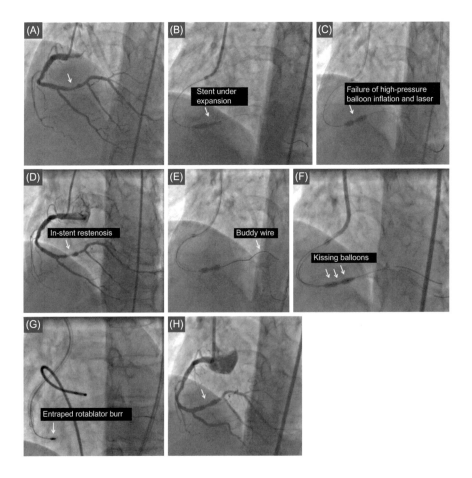

carry additional risks. For example, rotational atherectomy has been successfully used to expand an underexpanded stent ("stentablation"),[12−14] but may result in stent material or plaque embolization, burr entrapment (Figure 9.2), and stent damage necessitating implantation of an additional stent.[13] Laser can help expand an underexpanded stent[8] but carries risk for perforation, especially if contrast is simultaneously injected. Similarly, use of cutting balloon or Angiosculpt may be complicated by fracture of the cutting balloon blade,[15] stent strut avulsion,[16,17] and balloon entrapment.[18−20]

References

1. Raja Y, Routledge HC, Doshi SN. A noncompliant, high pressure balloon to manage undilatable coronary lesions. *Catheter Cardiovasc Interv* 2010;**75**:1067−73.
2. Yazdanfar S, Ledley GS, Alfieri A, Strauss C, Kotler MN. Parallel angioplasty dilatation catheter and guide wire: a new technique for the dilatation of calcified coronary arteries. *Cathet Cardiovasc Diagn* 1993;**28**:72−5.

◀ **Figure 9.2 Case example of a stented "balloon undilatable" lesion.** A 64-year-old man presented with non-ST segment elevation acute myocardial infarction and was found to have a left anterior descending artery culprit lesion that was stented. He also had a lesion in the posterolateral vessel (PLV) that was directly stented; however, the stent balloon did not expand (arrow, B). Multiple high-pressure balloon inflations and laser were performed without success in expanding the stent (arrow, C). The patient returned a few months later with recurrent chest pain and significant in-stent restenosis of the "balloon undilatable" lesion was noted (arrow, D). Repeat dilation with a non-compliant balloon and a buddy wire (arrow, E) and with kissing balloons (arrows, F) was performed without success. Rotational atherectomy was complicated by burr entrapment (arrow, G; note deep guide catheter engagement), resulting in loss of distal flow and hemodynamic instability requiring intraaortic balloon pump insertion. The burr was successfully removed, but stent underexpansion persisted (arrow, H).
Source: Courtesy of Dr. Elizabeth Holper.

3. Stillabower ME. Longitudinal force focused coronary angioplasty: a technique for resistant lesions. *Cathet Cardiovasc Diagn* 1994;**32**:196−8.
4. Meerkin D. My buddy, my friend: focused force angioplasty using the buddy wire technique in an inadequately expanded stent. *Catheter Cardiovasc Interv* 2005;**65**:513−5.
5. Lindsey JB, Banerjee S, Brilakis ES. Two "buddies" may be better than one: use of two buddy wires to expand an underexpanded left main coronary stent. *J Invasive Cardiol* 2007;**19**:E355−8.
6. Wilson A, Ardehali R, Brinton TJ, Yeung AC, Lee DP. Cutting balloon inflation for drug-eluting stent underexpansion due to unrecognized coronary arterial calcification. *Cardiovasc Revasc Med* 2006;**7**:185−8.
7. Pappy R, Gautam A, Abu-Fadel MS. AngioSculpt PTCA balloon catheter entrapment and detachment managed with stent jailing. *J Invasive Cardiol* 2010;**22**:E208−10.
8. Ben-Dor I, Maluenda G, Pichard AD, et al. The use of excimer laser for complex coronary artery lesions. *Cardiovasc Revasc Med* 2011;**12** (69):e1−8.
9. Fernandez JP, Hobson AR, McKenzie D, et al. Beyond the balloon: excimer coronary laser atherectomy used alone or in combination with rotational atherectomy in the treatment of chronic total occlusions, non-crossable and non-expansible coronary lesions. *EuroIntervention* 2013;**9**:243−50.
10. Badr S, Ben-Dor I, Dvir D, et al. The state of the excimer laser for coronary intervention in the drug-eluting stent era. *Cardiovasc Revasc Med* 2013;**14**:93−8.
11. Sunew J, Chandwaney RH, Stein DW, Meyers S, Davidson CJ. Excimer laser facilitated percutaneous coronary intervention of a nondilatable coronary stent. *Catheter Cardiovasc Interv* 2001;**53**:513−7 [discussion 8]
12. Kobayashi Y, Teirstein P, Linnemeier T, Stone G, Leon M, Moses J. Rotational atherectomy (stent ablation) in a lesion with stent underexpansion due to heavily calcified plaque. *Catheter Cardiovasc Interv* 2001;**52**:208−11.
13. Medina A, de Lezo JS, Melian F, Hernandez E, Pan M, Romero M. Successful stent ablation with rotational atherectomy. *Catheter Cardiovasc Interv* 2003;**60**:501−4.
14. Fournier JA, Florian F, Ballesteros SM. Rotational atherectomy of a lesion in which stent expansion was limited by severe calcification. *Rev Esp Cardiol* 2005;**58**:879−80.

15. Haridas KK, Vijayakumar M, Viveka K, Rajesh T, Mahesh NK. Fracture of cutting balloon microsurgical blade inside coronary artery during angioplasty of tough restenotic lesion: a case report. *Catheter Cardiovasc Interv* 2003;**58**:199−201.
16. Harb TS, Ling FS. Inadvertent stent extraction six months after implantation by an entrapped cutting balloon. *Catheter Cardiovasc Interv* 2001;**53**:415−9.
17. Wang HJ, Kao HL, Liau CS, Lee YT. Coronary stent strut avulsion in aorto-ostial in-stent restenosis: potential complication after cutting balloon angioplasty. *Catheter Cardiovasc Interv* 2002;**56**:215−9.
18. Kawamura A, Asakura Y, Ishikawa S, et al. Extraction of previously deployed stent by an entrapped cutting balloon due to the blade fracture. *Catheter Cardiovasc Interv* 2002;**57**:239−43.
19. Sanchez-Recalde A, Galeote G, Martin-Reyes R, Moreno R. AngioSculpt PTCA balloon entrapment during dilatation of a heavily calcified lesion. *Rev Esp Cardiol* 2008;**61**:1361−3.
20. Giugliano GR, Cox N, Popma J. Cutting balloon entrapment during treatment of in-stent restenosis: an unusual complication and its management. *J Invasive Cardiol* 2005;**17**:168−70.

10 Radiation Management During CTO PCI

Radiation skin injury (Figure 10.1) is a rare complication of any invasive cardiac procedure but is more likely to occur in the setting of complex procedures, such as chronic total occlusion (CTO) percutaneous coronary intervention (PCI). Radiation injury can lead to severe consequences for the **patient**, such as painful, non-healing ulcers, that may require months or even years to heal, sometimes requiring surgical debridement and plastic reconstruction.

Radiation dose management from the outset of the case is essential. Best practices for dose reduction for the patient also reduce **physician and staff** dosing. Interventional cardiologists and staff are exposed to ionizing radiation on a daily basis over many years, which potentially predisposes to cancer (such as, but not limited to, left-sided brain tumors[2]), cataracts, and other ailments, as well as the comorbidities associated with protective garments.[3] However, despite the obvious benefits in limiting radiation exposure, observations from multiple cardiac catheterization laboratories have shown that sound radiation management practices are very infrequently implemented.[4] The goal of this chapter is to provide simple and practical tips and tricks for reducing both patient and operator radiation exposure.[1,5,6]

10.1 Why is Radiation Management Important?

1. To prevent radiation injury to the patient.
2. To prevent radiation injury to the operator and the cardiac laboratory staff.

Manual of Coronary Chronic Total Occlusion Interventions. DOI: http://dx.doi.org/10.1016/B978-0-12-420129-3.00010-6

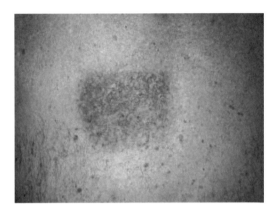

**Figure 10.1 Example of radiation-induced skin injury after CTO
PCI.** Erythema and epilation developed on a patient's back 1 month after
CTO PCI, during which he received 11.8 Gy air kerma dose.
Source: Reproduced with permission from Ref. 1.

3. To prevent medico-legal consequences, since significant radiation exposure (the threshold varies from state to state) is considered a sentinel
   event by the Joint Commission for Hospital Accreditation.
4. Because there is increasing public and medical community concern
   about radiation exposure during medical procedures, both regarding
   an individual procedure and the lifelong cumulative radiation exposure
   of patients.

10.2 Essentials of Radiation Dose Management

It is recommended that operators wishing to develop a CTO (or any
complex PCI) program consult with their institution radiation officers
to implement strict radiation management protocols and safe radiation management practices.

> There are two ways to minimize radiation during CTO PCI
> procedures:
>
> 1. By acquiring the skillsets and expertise to perform safe and efficient
>   CTO PCI procedures (as described throughout this manual).
> 2. By implementing safe radiation management practices.

The rest of this chapter focuses on radiation management practices.

1. **Dose assessment: Understand how radiation is measured in the cardiac cath lab and which radiation measure should be looked at.**

    Assessment of radiation dose in the cardiac cath lab is much more than fluoroscopy time (FT, measured in minutes). With several limitations, the most obvious of which is its failure to include cine imaging, FT alone is not adequate to assess patient radiation dose. The actual administered radiation dose depends on multiple other factors, such as the weight of the patient, the use of collimation, the positioning of the table and image intensifier, and the imaging angles. For this reason, since 2006 all fluoroscopic equipment sold in the United States have additional parameters to identify patient dose measured, recorded, and displayed during the procedure.

    There are currently two standard parameters reported on interventional fluoroscopic equipment: total **air kerma** (AK) at the interventional reference point (measured in Gray (Gy)) and **dose area product** (DAP, measured in Gycm^2) (Figure 10.2). DAP is used to monitor the potential for

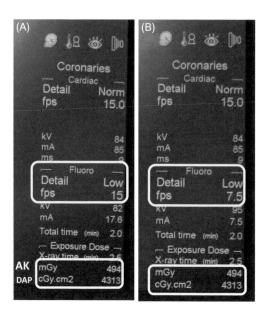

Figure 10.2 Screenshot from a GE (General Electric) X-ray machine screen, highlighting the fluoroscopy frames per second (yellow box: 15 fps in A versus 7.5 fps in B). Also, the air kerma (494 mGy or 0.494 Gy) and the DAP radiation dose are highlighted.

genetic defects or cancer risk over time (called *stochastic effects*) and is not used for intraprocedural radiation dose monitoring.

The air kerma dose is the dose that the CTO operator should constantly monitor to determine the risk that the patient will develop radiation skin injury and to adjust the procedural plan. Total **air kerma** is the procedural cumulative X-ray energy delivered to air at the interventional reference point, i.e., 15 cm on the X-ray tube side of isocenter—the point at which the primary X-ray beam intersects with the rotational axis of the C-arm gantry.[1] Kerma stands for *K*inetic *E*nergy *R*eleased in *Ma*tter. Although the **air kerma** dose is an approximation of the actual radiation that the patient receives during a procedure, it is a far better and physiologically relevant index compared to FT. The **air kerma dose** directly correlates with the risk of radiation skin injury, which is called *deterministic effects* (Figure 10.1).

The following air kerma dose thresholds are important to remember:[3]

> **5 Gy**: Below this threshold skin injury is unlikely to occur.
> **10 Gy**: Skin injury is likely, requiring physicist assessment of the case.
> **15 Gy**: This is considered a sentinel event by the Joint Commission for Hospital Accreditation and requires reporting to the regulatory authorities in the United States.

---

2. Laboratory environment

All cardiac cath labs should have a radiation safety program with active participation of physicians, staff, and physicists. All interventional cardiologists should apply two basic principles of radiation protection to their practice: reduce radiation exposure to "as low as reasonably achievable" (**ALARA**) and ensure procedure **justification**, such that no patient receives radiation without potential benefit.

Although only certain states mandate fluoroscopy training, it is important that everyone receives radiation dose management and safety training commensurate to their responsibilities. The National Council on Radiation Protection recommends both didactic and hands-on training. The didactic program should include initial training with periodic updates covering the topics of radiation physics and safety. Hands-on training should be provided for newly hired operators and all operators on newly purchased equipment.

It is the individual's responsibility to wear a dosimeter. Although a single dosimeter worn outside the collar can be used, two properly worn dosimeters—one at waist under and one at collar outside the protective garment—provide a better reflection of effective dose. Protective garments stop approximately 95% of the scatter radiation. Radiation glasses are effective but must fit properly and have 0.25-mm lead equivalent protection and additional side shielding. Ceiling-mounted and below-table shielding are also effective; both should be used routinely.

Current fluoroscopic X-ray systems offer features for dose management including frame-rate adjustment, virtual collimation, last image hold, X-ray store, and real-time dose display. Image quality is a function of multiple patient, procedure, and equipment variables. As a general rule, image quality and radiation dose are tightly woven. Automatic dose rate controls increase dose for a specific patient size in a specific projection to achieve adequate image quality. Knowing the equipment and working with a qualified physicist are essential for dose optimization.

3. Procedure-based radiation dose management

Table 10.1 provides a procedure-based dose management outline. Preprocedure planning is an essential component to radiation dose management. It is important to detect factors that place patients at high risk for radiation-induced skin injury, such as obesity or recent fluoroscopic procedures within the previous 30–60 days. Informed consent for CTO PCI should include radiation safety information.

The following tips and tricks can assist with intraprocedural radiation dose management:

A. Carefully monitor radiation exposure throughout the procedure.

The operator should consider stopping the procedure if 12 Gy air kerma dose is administered without the procedure nearly completed, or if 7–10 Gy is reached without crossing the CTO. It is recommended that each cath lab have a protocol for alerting the operator on radiation, e.g., announcing the dose used every 1000 mGy and/or every 30 min.

B. Do NOT place your hands in the direct radiation beam!!!

Operator and staff must maximize their distance from the X-ray tube (i.e., the inverse square law), which is of particular importance for radial access cases. All appendages—operators' and patients'—should be out of the imaging field!

If there are challenges while obtaining access, it is best to remove the operator's hands from the directly imaged field, while X-ray imaging is on (Figure 10.3). A device was recently introduced to

Table 10.1 Procedure-Based Case Management of Radiation Dose

I. Preprocedure
  A. Radiation safety program for catheterization laboratory
    1. Dosimeter use, shielding, training/education
  B. Imaging equipment and operator knowledge
    1. On-screen dose assessment (air kerma, DAP)
    2. Dose saving: store fluoroscopy, adjustable pulse and frame rate, and last image hold
  C. Preprocedure dose planning
    1. Assess patient and procedure, including patient's size and lesion(s) complexity
  D. Informed patient with appropriate consent
II. Procedure
  A. Limit fluoroscopy: step on petal only when looking at screen
  B. Limit cine: store fluoroscopy when image quality not required
  C. Limit magnification, frame rate, steep angles
  D. Use collimation and filters to fullest extent possible
  E. Vary tube angle when possible to change skin area exposed
  F. Position table and image receptor: X-ray tube too close to patient increases dose; high image receptor increases scatter
  G. Keep patient and operator body parts out of field of view
  H. Maximize shielding and distance from X-ray source for all personnel
  I. Manage and monitor dose in real time from beginning of case
III. Postprocedure
  A. Document radiation dose in records (FT, $K_{a,r}$, P_{KA})
  B. Notify patient and referring physician when high dose delivered
    1. $K_{a,r} > 5$ Gy, chart document; inform patient; arrange follow-up
    2. $K_{a,r} > 10$ Gy, qualified physicist should calculate skin dose
    3. PSD > 15 Gy, Joint Commission sentinel event
  C. Assess and refer adverse skin effects to appropriate consultant

Abbreviations: $K_{a,r}$ = total air kerma at reference point; P_{KA} = air kerma area product; PSD = peak skin dose.
Source: Modified from Ref. 1.

allow obtaining access while keeping the physician's hands away from the peak radiation zone during puncture (Quick-Access Needle Holder, Spectranetics, Figure 10.4). It is also important to exclude from the radiation field the patient's arm, since it increases the radiation delivered, as well as the risk of radiation injury to the patient's upper extremity.

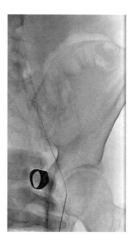

Figure 10.3 Example of what should NOT be done while obtaining access (i.e., placing the hand under the direct X-ray beam).
Source: Reproduced with permission from HMP Communications.[4]

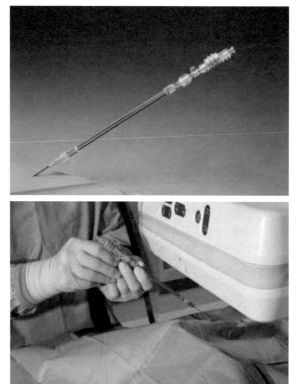

Figure 10.4 Image of quick-access needle holder.
Source: Reproduced with permission from Spectranetics.

C. Minimize fluoroscopy frame rate.

Most modern X-ray equipment (GE, Toshiba, Siemens, Shimadzu, and Phillips) allows the operator to change the fluoroscopy frames per second (fps). Most machines default to 15 fps for cardiac procedures. Decreasing the fluoroscopy fps from 15 to 7.5 fps (Figure 10.2) cuts fluoroscopy-related radiation in half. Although the images obtained at 7.5 fps are less pristine than those obtained at 15 fps, they are perfectly adequate for most, if not all, CTO PCI maneuvers. Many operators currently use 7.5 fps fluoroscopy for all cardiac procedures, not just CTO PCI. It is easiest for operators to get familiar with the 7.5 fps mode during conventional PCI procedures before adopting this practice in the more complex CTO PCI procedures.

D. Do NOT step on the fluoroscopy pedal when not looking at the screen.

Although this appears self-evident, it is amazing how often this simple principle is ignored! There is high prevalence of the "heavy foot" syndrome, i.e., continuing to perform fluoroscopy when it is not needed!

E. Use techniques that limit fluoroscopy.

An example is the "trapping" technique for over-the-wire equipment exchanges, regardless of whether short or long (300 cm) wires are used (Section 3.7). Another example is using a torquer to mark the length of the wire that can be safely advanced through a microcatheter without exiting into the vessel, obviating the need for fluoroscopy during this maneuver.

F. Use techniques that limit cine-angiography.

Cine-angiography exposes the patient to $10\times$ higher dose compared to fluoroscopy and is not reflected in the FT. The "image store" or "fluoro save" function is available in most modern X-ray equipment and should be used instead of cine to document balloon and stent inflations. Also, when performing dual injection (Section 3.2), the CTO collateral donor vessel can be injected before starting cine recording, as it takes time for the contrast to fill the CTO distal true lumen.

G. Use of low magnification.

Lower magnification requires less radiation exposure. Similar to using 7.5 fps, using lower magnification requires a "learning curve" to adjust to the change in image quality. Some X-ray equipment (Toshiba) has software for "virtual magnification," which allows for images obtained in low magnification to be magnified and displayed on the screen as larger images. Although the angiographic definition using this method is somewhat less sharp, it is still adequate for most cases.

H. Use collimation.

Collimation reduces the size of the skin area exposed to radiation and reduces the overall dose received by the patient. A caveat of collimation is that some equipment (e.g., the tips of guidewires or guide catheters) may not be included in the field of view, requiring intermittent monitoring to ensure that no significant changes have occurred (e.g., excessive distal migration of a guidewire that can lead to distal vessel perforation or deep engagement of the guide catheter that can lead to aortocoronary dissection).

I. Frequently rotate the image intensifier to minimize the exposure of each area of the skin.

Using multiple angles during fluoroscopy and cine-angiography is critical during long procedures to minimize radiation exposure to the same skin entry point. High radiation dose may not be as deleterious if it is applied to multiple areas of skin, because the dose to each particular area is reduced.

J. Optimize the position of the table (as high as possible) and the image intensifier (as close to the patient as possible) (Figure 10.5).

K. Avoid steep angles of the image intensifier.

Since steep angles are associated with higher radiation exposure due to penetration through more tissue, less steep angles are preferred. The anteroposterior may, however, not be the optimal projection, because the spine is included in the field. The right anterior oblique projection can result in less radiation exposure but can be challenging for mid right coronary artery wiring, although it is excellent for wiring septal collaterals or working in the mid left anterior descending artery.

L. Use the X-ray stand position memory.

X-ray machines can store multiple stand positions in memory and can automatically move to a selected position on command. This enables the operator to avoid the use of fluoroscopy to achieve a desired stand position; however, this might increase the dose of the X-ray to two or more skin areas under the exact same angles stored in the memory.[7]

M. Use of radiation-monitoring devices that provide real-time feedback on operator radiation exposure.

An example of such a device is shown in Figure 10.6.

N. Use additional shielding.

In addition to standard ceiling-attached and personal lead protection, adding a 1.0-mm lead flap below the lead glass and lead top along the undercouch lead shield (Figure 10.7) can effectively reduce

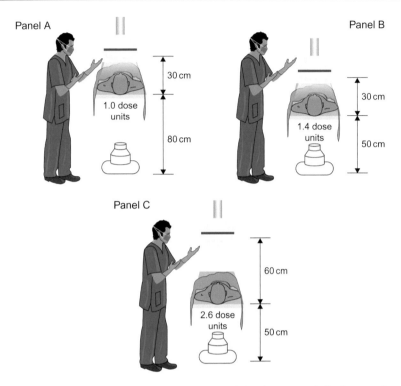

Figure 10.5 Example of optimal table positioning to minimize patient (and operator) radiation exposure. Panel A: the physician performs the procedure with the patient table elevated and the image intensifier close to the patient (total distance from the X-ray tube to the detector = 110 cm). Panel B: the physician employs a lower table setting but maintains the image intensifier close to the patient's chest (total distance from the X-ray tube to the detector = 80 cm). Because of the closer proximity to the X-ray tube, the dose rate to the patient at the beam entrance port will be about 40% higher. Panel C: the physician employs a low table height but has elevated the image intensifier (total distance from the X-ray tube to the detector = 110 cm). The skin dose to the patient on panel C is 260% that of the patient on panel A. (The image generated by the configuration on panel C is 40−50% larger owing to geometric magnification caused by the elevated image intensifier.) If the procedure on panel A required a 3-Gy skin dose, the same procedure employing the panel B configuration would result in a 4.2-Gy dose, whereas the one performed employing the configuration on panel C would result in 7.8-Gy dose.
Source: Reproduced with permission from Ref. 7.

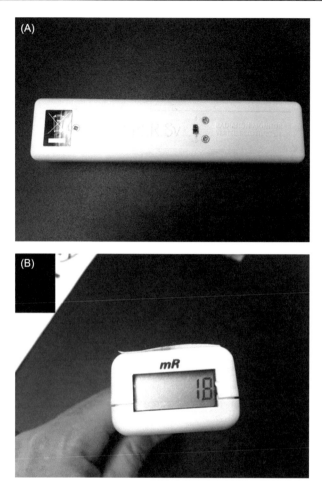

Figure 10.6 Example of a radiation-monitoring device that provides real-time auditory feedback to the operator on the level of radiation exposure.

radiation exposure to the operator to <1% of typical levels by reducing scatter leakages.

Moreover, additional shielding can be placed in the sterile field to reduce scatter radiation, such as the RadPad shields (Worldwide Innovations & Technologies) (Section 2.10) (which should be placed over the patient's abdomen).

New radiation protection systems, such as the Zero Gravity (CFI Medical Solutions, Fenton, MI) and the Trinity Radiation Protection System[9] can further reduce or eliminate operator radiation exposure, while also obviating the adverse orthopedic consequences of wearing lead aprons.

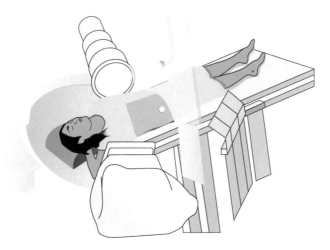

Figure 10.7 Position of undercouch top, flap below the glass sheet, and lead shield on the patient's abdomen.
Source: Reproduced with permission from Ref. 8.

O. Always examine the patient's back prior to starting a CTO PCI procedure.

Patients with coronary CTOs often have had multiple prior diagnostic or interventional procedures. They tend to have extensive atherosclerotic disease and may have had several prior non-CTO PCIs. In large CTO referral centers it is not uncommon to treat patients with previously failed CTO PCI attempts that might have resulted in large amounts of radiation exposure. Performing a CTO PCI procedure in a patient with an unrecognized preexisting radiation burn can be catastrophic.

P. For patients with prior radiation-induced skin injury that need repeat procedures.

Among patients with prior radiation-induced dermatitis, avoidance of repeat exposure is preferred although it may be unavoidable in selected clinical circumstances. In such instances, methods to avoid and/or limit focal radiation exposure to the injured site are essential. A radiation shield may be constructed from a commercially available shielding product (RadPad, Worldwide Innovations & Technologies). Specifically, the shield is tailored to the area of skin injury by cutting the shield and placing it over the skin at the site of previous injury (Figure 10.8A and B). The shield will attenuate approximately 90% of direct beam radiation and permit a visible "shade" to the operator under fluoroscopic guidance that obscures visualization and requires alteration of the beam angle.

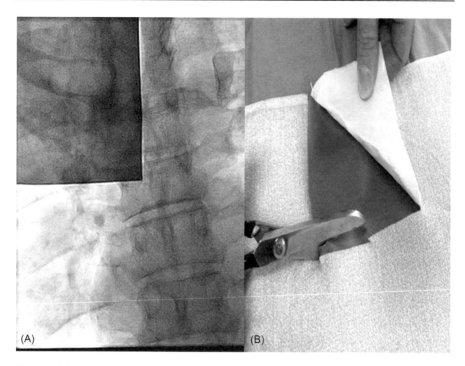

Figure 10.8 Example of a technique for performing repeat cardiac catheterization among patients with prior skin radiation injury. A piece of a radiation shield is cut out (B) in the shape of the prior radiation injury skin area and placed over the injured skin area (dark area on fluoroscopy as shown in A) to minimize radiation exposure of the same area.
Source: Courtesy of Dr. Karmpaliotis.

4. Postprocedure: follow-up and treatment

Cardiac catheterization reports should include all available radiation parameters: FT, air kerma dose, and DAP. Patient notification, chart documentation, and communication with the primary care provider should routinely occur following procedures with high radiation dose.

Patients Who Receive >5 Gy Air Kerma Dose Should Be Counseled About the Possibility of Radiation-Induced Skin Injury on Their Back

All patients who receive >5 Gy air kerma dose should be followed up within a month. During physical examination, the back of the patients should be inspected to detect any radiation injury; if such an injury is diagnosed, patients should be referred to specialists (dermatologist, plastic surgeons) for further evaluation and treatment. This is critical because if the patient is not aware of this risk and develops erythema and local discomfort (Figure 10.1), he or she may see a dermatologist who may biopsy the lesion, potentially leading to a non-healing ulcer.

For >10 Gy air kerma dose, a qualified physicist should promptly calculate peak skin dose and the patient's skin should be examined at 2−4 weeks.

The Joint Commission identifies peak skin doses >15 Gy as a sentinel event; hospital risk management and regulatory agencies need to be contacted within 24 h.

10.3 Conclusions

Starting a CTO PCI program is a great opportunity to improve our "radiation reducing" habits for all cardiac procedures. We strongly believe that radiation safety should be a top priority of a successful CTO PCI program. Once the appropriate routines are engrained, they become second nature and one performs them automatically.[4]

Radiation reduction is a win−win situation for both the patient and the operator. Investing the time and effort required to develop sound radiation reducing habits can provide high dividends for patients, physicians, and X-ray technicians.[4]

The interventional cardiologist performing CTO PCI, as the person responsible for all aspects of patient care in the cath lab, must be actively involved in managing radiation dose to maximize patient and staff safety. Roentgen died from radiation-induced cancer because he did not know the devastating consequences of X-ray exposure. We do not have the same excuse: We should never forget that being unable to see an immediate effect of radiation on our body or the patients' bodies does not mean that we are safe.[4]

References

1. Chambers CE. Radiation dose in percutaneous coronary intervention OUCH did that hurt? *JACC Cardiovasc Interv* 2011;**4**:344−6.
2. Roguin A, Goldstein J, Bar O, Goldstein JA. Brain and neck tumors among physicians performing interventional procedures. *Am J Cardiol* 2013;**111**:1368−72.

3. Klein LW, Miller DL, Balter S, et al. Occupational health hazards in the interventional laboratory: time for a safer environment. *Catheter Cardiovasc Interv* 2009;**73**:432–8.
4. Brilakis ES, Patel VG. What you can't see can hurt you! *J Invasive Cardiol* 2012;**24**:421.
5. Chambers CE, Fetterly KA, Holzer R, et al. Radiation safety program for the cardiac catheterization laboratory. *Catheter Cardiovasc Interv* 2011;**77**:546–56.
6. Fetterly KA, Lennon RJ, Bell MR, Holmes Jr. DR, Rihal CS. Clinical determinants of radiation dose in percutaneous coronary interventional procedures: influence of patient size, procedure complexity, and performing physician. *JACC Cardiovasc Interv* 2011;**4**:336–43.
7. Hirshfeld Jr. JW, Balter S, Brinker JA, et al. ACCF/AHA/HRS/SCAI clinical competence statement on physician knowledge to optimize patient safety and image quality in fluoroscopically guided invasive cardiovascular procedures. A report of the American College of Cardiology Foundation/American Heart Association/American College of Physicians Task Force on Clinical Competence and Training. *J Am Coll Cardiol* 2004;**44**:2259–82.
8. Kuon E, Schmitt M, Dahm JB. Significant reduction of radiation exposure to operator and staff during cardiac interventions by analysis of radiation leakage and improved lead shielding. *Am J Cardiol* 2002;**89**:44–9.
9. Fattal P, Goldstein JA. A novel complete radiation protection system eliminates physician radiation exposure and leaded aprons. *Catheter Cardiovasc Interv* 2013;**82**:11–6.

11 Stenting of CTO Lesions

11.1 Stent Type

Restenosis rates after chronic total occlusion (CTO) stenting can be relatively high. Bare metal stents (BMS) significantly reduce restenosis compared to balloon angioplasty alone,[1] yet the incidence of restenosis and re-occlusion remains very high. In the Total Occlusion Study of Canada 1 (TOSCA-1) trial, the 6-month incidence of restenosis and re-occlusion with BMS exceeded 50% and 10%, respectively.[2]

First generation drug-eluting stents (DES) significantly reduced restenosis compared to BMS. The first randomized-controlled trial comparing BMS and DES was the Primary Stenting of Totally Occluded Native Coronary Arteries (**PRISON II**) trial that compared BMS with the sirolimus-eluting stent (SES, Cypher, Cordis). The SES significantly reduced the 6-month incidence of binary angiographic restenosis (from 41% to 11%, $p < 0.001$), vessel re-occlusion (from 13% to 4%, $p < 0.04$), and the need for new revascularization procedures (from 22% to 8%, $p < 0.001$) compared to BMS.[3] The benefit persisted at 5-year follow-up angiography, although some late catch-up in lumen diameter loss was observed in the SES group.[4] Two other studies, the Gruppo Italiano di Studio sullo Stent nelle Occlusioni Coronariche Societá Italiana di Cardiologia Invasiva (**GISSOC II-GISE**)[5] and the **CORACTO** trial,[6] showed similar results. Four meta-analyses on first generation DES versus BMS in CTOs were published in 2010−2011,[7−10] all reporting significant reduction in the risk for restenosis, re-occlusion, and repeat revascularization with DES. DES appeared to be safe in CTOs, although the risk for stent thrombosis was higher with DES in one meta-analysis.[7]

Second generation DES have been shown to provide incremental benefit compared to the first generation paclitaxel-eluting stent in

Manual of Coronary Chronic Total Occlusion Interventions. DOI: http://dx.doi.org/10.1016/B978-0-12-420129-3.00011-8

non-CTO lesions.[11] Three randomized clinical trials have compared the first generation SES with the second generation everolimus-eluting stent (EES, Xience V, Abbott Vascular)[12] and zotarolimus-eluting stent (ZES, Medtronic)[13] in CTOs. The Chronic Coronary Occlusion Treated by Everolimus-Eluting Stent (**CIBELES**) compared EES with SES and demonstrated similar restenosis and repeat revascularization rates, with a trend for lower stent thrombosis risk in the EES group (3% versus 0%, $p = 0.075$). The Catholic Total Occlusion Study (**CATOS**) trial showed similar angiographic and clinical outcomes with the SES and the Endeavor ZES (Medtronic).[13] In contrast, the **PRISON III** trial reported higher in-segment late lumen loss at 8-month follow-up angiography with the Endeavor ZES compared to the SES, although rates were similar with the Resolute ZES.[13] Finally, in an Italian registry of 802 patients undergoing CTO PCI over 8 years, use of EES was associated with a significantly lower re-occlusion rate compared to first generation DES (3.0% versus 10.1%, $p < 0.001$).[14]

As described in detail in Chapter 5, extensive dissection/re-entry crossing strategies (such as the subintimal tracking and re-entry— STAR—technique) are associated with high restenosis and re-occlusion rates and should only be used as a last resort.[14,15] Outcomes after limited dissection/re-entry have received limited study. Among 170 patients undergoing CTO PCI, use of the BridgePoint Medical system was associated with equally high success and equally low complication rates as other techniques, both immediately postprocedure and during long-term follow-up, in spite of its use in higher complexity cases.[16]

In patients with prior coronary bypass graft surgery, treatment of a native coronary artery CTO is preferable to treatment of a saphenous vein graft (SVG) CTO supplying the same territory, because of very high (>50%) restenosis rates after SVG CTO PCI.[17] Occasionally, occluded SVGs can be used as retrograde access to the native coronary artery CTO. If native CTO PCI is not possible, PCI of the SVG CTO may be a reasonable treatment option.[17−21]

In summary, second generation DES (EES and Resolute ZES) provide better outcomes compared to first generation DES and are currently the preferred options for CTO PCI. In the future, bioabsorbable scaffolds may further improve outcomes, as they could address a major limitation of metallic stents in CTOs, i.e., late-acquired malapposition, due to significant enlargement of the CTO target vessel after successful recanalization.[22]

11.2   Stent Optimization

Maximizing stent expansion is important for decreasing the risk for restenosis, which remains relatively high, even with second generation DES (approximately 10−15% at one year) and possibly stent thrombosis. Optimal stent expansion can be accomplished using the following techniques:

1. **Appropriate stent sizing**

   The CTO vessel often increases in size in the months following successful CTO PCI. In one study, 69% of the recanalized vessel had a mean increase in lumen diameter of 0.4 mm over a period of 6 months.[23] Intravascular imaging may help optimize stent sizing at the index procedure: stent undersizing can lead to stent malapposition and higher long-term restenosis and stent thrombosis rates, whereas stent oversizing may lead to perforation.

   Optical coherence tomography may also be very useful for selecting the optimum stent length and detecting areas of dissection that require stenting (Figure 11.1).[24]

   Overall, it is recommended to avoid stenting excessively long vessel segments, as longer stent length may increase the risk for restenosis and possibly stent thrombosis. This is frequently referred to as "mission creep," or the tendency to make the distal vessel look perfect, rather than just treating the CTO.

2. **High-pressure balloon inflation**

   High-pressure balloon inflations are critical for adequate stent expansion, especially in calcified vessels. Routine postdilation of

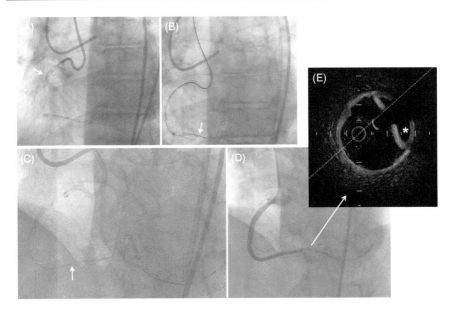

Figure 11.1 Example of distal dissection confirmed with optical coherence tomography. A right coronary artery CTO (arrow, A) was crossed subintimally using antegrade wire escalation (B). The Stingray system (arrow, C) was used, enabling successful re-entry into the distal true lumen, however, subsequent angiography demonstrated suboptimal distal result (D). Optical coherence tomography demonstrated a distal dissection with compression of the true lumen (asterisk, E) that was treated with implantation of an additional stent.

stents placed in CTOs should be performed using non-compliant balloons at high (20 atm or higher) pressures. However, high-pressure postdilation of oversized stents should be avoided, as it could lead to perforation.

3. Intravascular imaging

Intravascular imaging with intravascular ultrasonography (IVUS) or optical coherence tomography (OCT) can help detect areas of underexpansion, malapposition, or dissection (Figure 11.1), treatment of which may further improve outcomes of CTO PCI. OCT can be very useful in limiting the extent of stenting by confirming that the small caliber of the distal coronary vessel is due to chronic hypoperfusion and not due to dissection or atherosclerotic lesions.[22,24]

11.3 Antiplatelet Therapy After CTO Stenting

The optimal duration of dual antiplatelet therapy (DAPT) remains poorly defined: 12 months are currently recommended,[25] but many operators empirically recommend longer DAPT duration after CTO PCI in view of the often long stent lengths ("full metal jacket"), especially in the right coronary artery. Although 1- and 3-month DAPT durations have received Conformité Européenne (CE) mark after implantation of the Resolute ZES and the Xience EES, respectively, it remains unknown whether such short DAPT durations are safe in the context of CTO PCI. First generation DES appeared to have increased risk for stent thrombosis compared to BMS,[7] which has not been observed with second generation DES, especially EES.[12]

In summary, implantation of a second generation DES, ensuring good stent expansion and apposition, and at least 12 months of DAPT administration are critical for maximizing the likelihood of long-term patency after successful CTO recanalization.

References

1. Agostoni P, Valgimigli M, Biondi-Zoccai GG, et al. Clinical effectiveness of bare-metal stenting compared with balloon angioplasty in total coronary occlusions: insights from a systematic overview of randomized trials in light of the drug-eluting stent era. *Am Heart J* 2006;**151**:682−9.
2. Buller CE, Dzavik V, Carere RG, et al. Primary stenting versus balloon angioplasty in occluded coronary arteries: the Total Occlusion Study of Canada (TOSCA). *Circulation* 1999;**100**:236−42.
3. Suttorp MJ, Laarman GJ, Rahel BM, et al. Primary Stenting of Totally Occluded Native Coronary Arteries II (PRISON II): a randomized comparison of bare metal stent implantation with sirolimus-eluting stent implantation for the treatment of total coronary occlusions. *Circulation* 2006;**114**:921−8.
4. Teeuwen K, Van den Branden BJ, Rahel BM, et al. Late catch-up in lumen diameter at five-year angiography in MACE-free patients treated with sirolimus-eluting stents in the Primary Stenting of Totally Occluded Native Coronary Arteries: a randomised comparison of bare metal stent implantation with sirolimus-eluting stent implantation for the treatment of total coronary occlusions (PRISON II). *EuroIntervention* 2013;**9**:212−9.

5. Rubartelli P, Petronio AS, Guiducci V, et al. Comparison of sirolimus-eluting and bare metal stent for treatment of patients with total coronary occlusions: results of the GISSOC II-GISE multicentre randomized trial. *Eur Heart J* 2010;**31**:2014−20.

6. Reifart N, Hauptmann KE, Rabe A, Enayat D, Giokoglu K. Short and long term comparison (24 months) of an alternative sirolimus-coated stent with bioabsorbable polymer and a bare metal stent of similar design in chronic coronary occlusions: the CORACTO trial. *EuroIntervention* 2010;**6**:356−60.

7. Colmenarez HJ, Escaned J, Fernandez C, et al. Efficacy and safety of drug-eluting stents in chronic total coronary occlusion recanalization: a systematic review and meta-analysis. *J Am Coll Cardiol* 2010;**55**:1854−66.

8. Saeed B, Kandzari DE, Agostoni P, et al. Use of drug-eluting stents for chronic total occlusions: a systematic review and meta-analysis. *Catheter Cardiovasc Interv* 2011;**77**:315−32.

9. Niccoli G, Leo A, Giubilato S, et al. A meta-analysis of first-generation drug-eluting vs bare-metal stents for coronary chronic total occlusion: effect of length of follow-up on clinical outcome. *Int J Cardiol* 2011;**150**:351−4.

10. Ma J, Yang W, Singh M, Peng T, Fang N, Wei M. Meta-analysis of long-term outcomes of drug-eluting stent implantations for chronic total coronary occlusions. *Heart Lung* 2011;**40**:e32−40.

11. Kedhi E, Joesoef KS, McFadden E, et al. Second-generation everolimus-eluting and paclitaxel-eluting stents in real-life practice (COMPARE): a randomised trial. *Lancet* 2010;**375**:201−9.

12. Moreno R, Garcia E, Teles R, et al. Randomized comparison of sirolimus-eluting and everolimus-eluting coronary stents in the treatment of total coronary occlusions: results from the chronic coronary occlusion treated by everolimus-eluting stent randomized trial. *Circ Cardiovasc Interv* 2013;**6**:21−8.

13. Park HJ, Kim HY, Lee JM, et al. Randomized comparison of the efficacy and safety of zotarolimus-eluting stents vs. sirolimus-eluting stents for percutaneous coronary intervention in chronic total occlusion—CAtholic Total Occlusion Study (CATOS) trial. *Circ J* 2012;**76**:868−75.

14. Valenti R, Vergara R, Migliorini A, et al. Predictors of reocclusion after successful drug-eluting stent-supported percutaneous coronary intervention of chronic total occlusion. *J Am Coll Cardiol* 2013;**61**:545−50.

15. Kandzari DE, Grantham JA, Lombardi W, Thompson C. Not all subintimal chronic total occlusion revascularization is alike. *J Am Coll Cardiol* 2013;**61**:2570.

16. Mogabgab O, Patel VG, Michael TT, et al. Long-term outcomes with use of the Bridgepoint Medical System for the recanalization of coronary chronic total occlusions. *J Invasive Cardiol* 2013;**25**:579–85.

17. Brilakis ES, Banerjee S, Lombardi WL. Retrograde recanalization of native coronary artery chronic occlusions via acutely occluded vein grafts. *Catheter Cardiovasc Interv* 2010;**75**:109–13.

18. Sachdeva R, Uretsky BF. Retrograde recanalization of a chronic total occlusion of a saphenous vein graft. *Catheter Cardiovasc Interv* 2009;**74**:575–8.

19. Takano M, Yamamoto M, Mizuno K. A retrograde approach for the treatment of chronic total occlusion in a patient with acute coronary syndrome. *Int J Cardiol* 2007;**119**:e22–4.

20. Ho PC, Tsuchikane E. Improvement of regional ischemia after successful percutaneous intervention of bypassed native coronary chronic total occlusion: an application of the CART technique. *J Invasive Cardiol* 2008;**20**:305–8.

21. Brilakis ES, Grantham JA, Thompson CA, et al. The retrograde approach to coronary artery chronic total occlusions: a practical approach. *Catheter Cardiovasc Interv* 2012;**79**:3–19.

22. Galassi AR, Tomasello SD, Crea F, et al. Transient impairment of vasomotion function after successful chronic total occlusion recanalization. *J Am Coll Cardiol* 2012;**59**:711–8.

23. Park JJ, Chae IH, Cho YS, et al. The recanalization of chronic total occlusion leads to lumen area increase in distal reference segments in selected patients: an intravascular ultrasound study. *JACC Cardiovasc Interv* 2012;**5**:827–36.

24. Jaguszewski M, Guagliumi G, Landmesser U. Optical frequency domain imaging for guidance of optimal stenting in the setting of recanalization of chronic total occlusion. *J Invasive Cardiol* 2013;**25**:367–8.

25. Levine GN, Bates ER, Blankenship JC, et al. 2011 ACCF/AHA/SCAI Guideline for Percutaneous Coronary Intervention. A report of the American College of Cardiology Foundation/American Heart Association Task Force on Practice Guidelines and the Society for Cardiovascular Angiography and Interventions. *J Am Coll Cardiol* 2011;**58** e44–e122.

12 Complications

From all that has been discussed in the previous chapters of this book, the reader will have already realized that chronic total occlusion (CTO) interventions are among the most complex percutaneous coronary interventions (PCI). In this chapter, we perform a thorough review of coronary and non-coronary complications that may occur in the course of CTO PCI. Awareness of the potential complications constitutes the cornerstone of their prevention. Furthermore, the various alternative techniques for complication management will be discussed.

Complications of CTO PCI can be classified according to timing (as acute and long term) and according to location (cardiac coronary, cardiac non-coronary, and non-cardiac). The acute complications of CTO PCI are summarized in Figure 12.1.[1]

The frequency of acute outcomes of CTO PCI from a 2013 meta-analysis of 65 studies with 18,061 patients is shown in Table 12.1.[2]

12.1 Acute Complications

12.1.1 Acute Coronary Complications

12.1.1.1 Acute Vessel Closure

12.1.1.1.1 Donor Vessel Injury During Retrograde CTO PCI

Although, by definition, CTO signifies that the target vessel is occluded for greater than 3 months, CTO PCI can be complicated by injury of a collateral donor vessel instrumented for contralateral angiography or for the retrograde approach (Figure 12.2). This is one of the most serious complications of CTO PCI and requires prompt

Manual of Coronary Chronic Total Occlusion Interventions. DOI: http://dx.doi.org/10.1016/B978-0-12-420129-3.00012-X

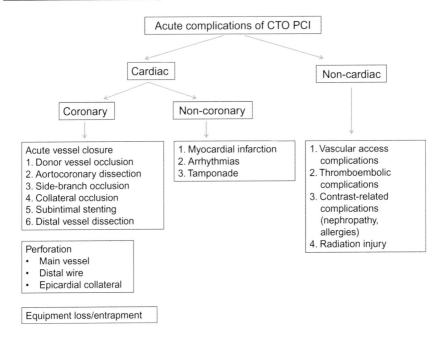

Figure 12.1 Classification of acute complications of CTO PCI.
Source: Modified with permission from Ref. 1.

identification and management, since it is frequently followed by extensive ischemia and hemodynamic decompensation. Unless this complication is rapidly and diligently treated with PCI or coronary artery bypass graft (CABG) surgery, it may result in death, particularly when the donor vessel is the last remaining vessel (a common situation in patients with prior CABG).[3]

Similar to planning of any PCI, a pretreatment plan should be in place in case donor vessel injury occurs. For example, when performing retrograde recanalization of the right coronary artery (RCA) in a patient with left main disease, pre-PCI intravascular ultrasound of the left main coronary artery is important. Similarly, intraaortic balloon pump availability is important when performing retrograde CTO PCI. In contrast to conventional PCI, management of donor vessel injury is complicated by the presence of hardware in the acutely occluded segment (microcatheters, externalized wires, etc.) that can hinder stenting as an emergency bailout solution.

Table 12.1 Frequency of Angiographic Success and Complications in CTO PCI

Outcome	Pooled Estimate Rate, %	95% CI	Reported Rate min, max %
Angiographic success	77.0	74.3–79.6	41.2–100.0
MACE	3.1	2.4–3.7	0–19.4
Death	0.2	0.1–0.3	0.0–3.6
Emergent CABG	0.1	0–0.2	0–2.3
Stroke	<0.01	0–0.1	0–0.7
Myocardial infarction	2.5	1.9–3.0	0–19.4
Q Wave myocardial infarction	0.2	0.1–0.3	0–2.6
Coronary perforation (per lesion)	2.9	2.2–3.6	0–11.9
Tamponade	0.3	0.2–0.5	0–4.7
Acute stent thrombosis	0.3	0.1–0.5	0–2.0
Vascular complication	0.6	0.3–0.9	0–2.8
Major bleed	0.4	0–0.7	0–3.7
Contrast nephropathy	3.8	2.4–5.3	2.4–18.1
Radiation skin injury	<0.01	0–0.1	0–11.1

CABG, coronary artery bypass graft surgery; MACE, major adverse cardiac events (composite of death, emergency CABG, stroke and myocardial infarction).
Modified with permission from[2].

Causes
a. **Catheter-induced vessel injury**. This may occur with either diagnostic or guide catheters, especially during equipment withdrawal that may cause the guide to deeply engage the vessel, or with forceful pulling of the snared retrograde guidewire.
b. Donor vessel thrombosis can occur during long procedures requiring coronary artery intubation by microcatheters or guidewires, especially when the level of anticoagulation is suboptimal (activated clotting time (ACT) <300 s).

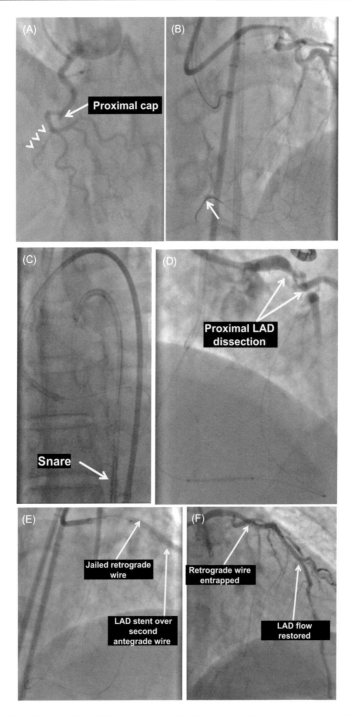

Figure 12.2 Example of donor vessel dissection during retrograde CTO PCI. PCI of an RCA CTO (A). After a failed antegrade crossing attempt,

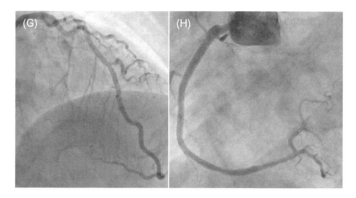

Figure 12.2 (Continued)

Prevention
a. Pay close attention to the position of diagnostic and guiding catheters (especially during equipment manipulations) and to the pressure waveform (dampening of the pressure waveform should be avoided and promptly corrected if it occurs). When dual injection is performed, the contralateral catheter should be removed as soon as it is not needed.
b. Never use a catheter with side holes to engage the CTO donor vessel, as it may mask suboptimal catheter position and flow compromise.
c. Maintain high ACT (the authors use >350 s for retrograde CTO PCI and >300 s for antegrade CTO PCI as discussed in section 3.5) to prevent donor vessel thrombosis. ACT checking should be performed every 20−30 min and should be delegated to a nurse, with a clear message that any drop in ACT below the pre-specified safety level should be communicated and corrected with additional boluses of unfractionated heparin.

◀ retrograde crossing was performed (B) and the retrograde guidewire was externalized (C). During RCA stenting over the externalized guidewire (D), the patient developed severe chest pain and hypotension due to proximal left anterior descending artery (LAD) dissection (D). The LAD was immediately stented (E) with restoration of antegrade flow and stabilization of the patient (F and G). After removal of the entrapped retrograde guidewire and stenting of the RCA, an excellent final angiographic result was achieved (H).

d. Avoid the retrograde approach through diffusely diseased donor vessels. Consider intracoronary imaging to investigate the anatomy of the donor vessel in advance. If the donor artery also requires PCI, it may be best treated on a separate setting before attempting retrograde CTO PCI.

e. Keep the retrograde guidewire encased by a microcatheter or over-the-wire balloon during all manipulations.[4]

f. Guidewire externalization leads to the creation of a wire loop with outstanding support for PCI devices, at the expense of communicating to the contralateral guiding catheter any traction during PCI, causing deep guide engagement and vessel damage. During externalization, meticulous attention should be paid to the contralateral catheter at all times.

g. Flush regularly all guiding and diagnostic catheters to prevent in-catheter thrombosis. Back-bleed the guide catheter after balloon trapping techniques are used to minimize the risk of air embolization.

h. Avoid use of the left internal mammary artery (LIMA) graft for retrograde CTO PCI because LIMA dissection can occur (Figure 12.3) and/or LIMA wiring may cause acute closure, if the LIMA tortuosity is straightened by the guidewire.[5]

i. Convert the retrograde system to a fully antegrade system either by using the kissing microcatheter technique[6] or by advancing a microcatheter over the retrograde wire into the distal vessel in an antegrade fashion and then exchanging the retrograde wire for an antegrade workhorse guidewire.

Treatment

a. Successful treatment of abrupt occlusion of the collateral donor artery becomes the highest priority of PCI. Treatment of the CTO should be aborted.

b. In anticipation of hemodynamic collapse, notify medical staff to prepare an intraaortic balloon pump, ensure femoral artery access (in radial procedures), prepare drugs, etc. while you concentrate in solving the abrupt occlusion.

c. Stenting is usually required to treat donor vessel dissections, as it is the fastest way to prevent its extension. If this complication occurs in the context of retrograde CTO PCI, the operator faces the problem of hardware in the donor vessel. Treatment options include:

    1. Withdrawing the retrograde wire, leaving the retrograde microcatheter beyond the acute occlusion, and exchanging for a regular PCI wire for stenting, avoiding the advancement of a new wire through a dissected segment.

    2. Using the externalized retrograde wire as a platform for stenting the acutely occluded donor vessel (provided it is anatomically feasible, e.g., in a short, limited dissection).

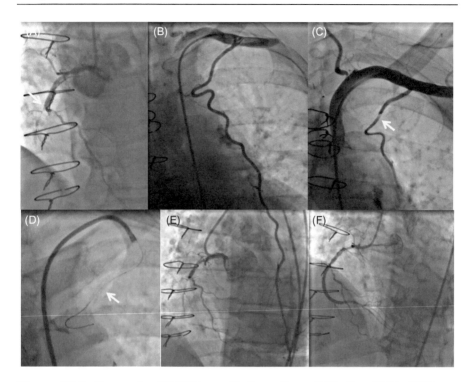

Figure 12.3 Example of LIMA graft dissection. PCI of an RCA CTO
(A) was attempted with dual injection via a catheter inserted in the LIMA
graft (B). Engagement of the LIMA graft was challenging due to an acute
takeoff angle. A Guideliner catheter was used to engage the LIMA causing
ostial LIMA dissection with decreased antegrade flow (C). LIMA flow was
restored after stenting (D), enabling continuation of the procedure (E), with
a final successful outcome (F).

3. Performing PCI with a second wire, jailing the externalized retrograde
   wire with the stent (Figure 12.2).
   Options 2 and 3 are more likely to be followed if CTO PCI is virtually completed (pending only CTO stenting, for example), while
   option 1 is probably the best choice if the CTO has not yet been
   crossed. Option 3 requires great caution during withdrawal of the
   jailed retrograde wire through the collateral channels (it may require
   protection with an antegrade microcatheter). An overall assessment of
   the patient's safety is mandatory at the time of deciding the best possible choice (e.g., contralateral femoral artery access may be required
   for intraaortic balloon pump insertion, making option 1 the preferred
   option).

d. Aspiration of thrombus and administration of glycoprotein IIb/IIIa inhibitors may be needed for donor vessel thrombosis. The ACT should be checked, as thrombosis may occur in other locations of the instrumented collateral donor vessel or the CTO target vessel.

12.1.1.1.2 Aortocoronary Dissection

Aortocoronary dissection is a rare complication which can occur with any PCI but is more common with CTO PCI (especially retrograde procedures) and most commonly occurs in the RCA[7] (Figures 12.4 and 12.5). Dissection may be limited to the coronary sinus but may extend to the proximal ascending aorta or even beyond the ascending aorta.[8]

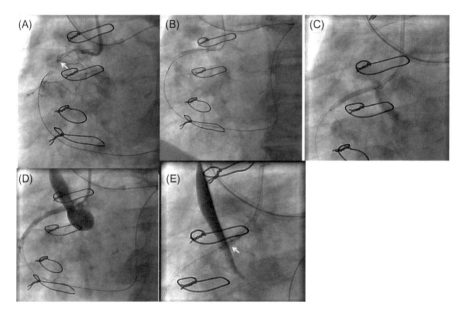

Figure 12.4 Illustration of an aortocoronary dissection during retrograde CTO intervention. Retrograde CTO intervention was performed to recanalize a proximal RCA CTO (arrow, A), using the reverse CART technique (B). Staining of the aortocoronary junction was observed with test injections during stent placement (C) that expanded when cine angiography was performed (D). Stenting of the RCA ostium was performed (arrow, E) without further antegrade contrast injections. The patient had an uneventful recovery. This case illustrates the importance of stopping antegrade contrast injections and stenting the vessel ostium if aortocoronary dissection occurs, in order to seal the dissection flap at the entry point of the dissection.
Source: Courtesy of Dr. Parag Doshi.

Prevention
a. Consider using anchor techniques (Section 3.6.5) as an alternative to aggressive guiding catheter intubation to enhance guide catheter support.
b. Use of guide catheters with side holes in occluded RCAs significantly decreases the risk of barotrauma. However, side-hole guide catheters may provide a false sense of security, as the pressure waveform may appear normal although aortocoronary dissection can still occur.
c. Power injectors should also be avoided or used with caution after the proximal segment of the CTO vessel has been dilated; manual injections are preferred.

Causes
a. Deep coronary engagement and utilization of aggressive guide catheters, such as 8 Fr Amplatz catheters.
b. Forceful contrast injection, especially through "wedged" guide catheters with dampened pressure waveform.
c. Predilation of the coronary ostium.
d. Balloon rupture.

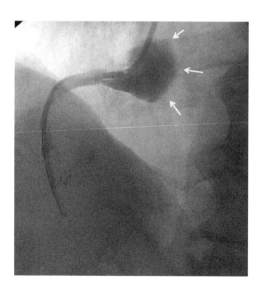

Figure 12.5 Example of aortocoronary dissection during antegrade CTO intervention. Aortocoronary dissection during attempts to cross an RCA CTO. The procedure was stopped and the patient had an uneventful recovery. Transesophageal echocardiography the following day demonstrated resolution of the dissection.
Source: Modified with permission from Ref. 1.

e. Retrograde wire advancement into the subintimal and subaortic space during the reverse controlled antegrade and retrograde tracking and dissection (CART) procedure.

Treatment
a. Stop injecting contrast into the coronary (as injections can expand the dissection plane).
b. Stent the ostium of the dissected coronary artery (with the stent protruding 1 mm into the aorta) to "seal" the dissection.
c. Use intravascular ultrasonography to guide stent placement and ensure complete ostial coverage.[9]
d. If the aortocoronary dissection is large, perform serial non-invasive imaging (with computed tomography or transesophageal echocardiography) to ensure that the dissection has stabilized and resolved. This is of particular importance if the dissection involves the ascending aorta.
e. Emergency surgery is rarely needed except in patients who develop aortic regurgitation, tamponade due to rupture into the pericardium, or extension of the dissection (Figure 12.6).[7,10]

12.1.1.1.3 Side-Branch Occlusion
Side-branch occlusion can occur during CTO PCI, especially when subintimal dissection/re-entry strategies are used, and is associated with higher frequency of post-PCI myocardial infarction (Figure 12.7).[7,11]

Causes
a. Use of dissection/re-entry strategies in vessels with side branches at the proximal or distal CTO cap.

Prevention
a. When treating CTOs that involve a bifurcation (e.g., those involving the RCA crux), a careful analysis of collateral support should be performed before the procedure, to determine whether both branches have independent collateral support.
b. Avoid use of (antegrade or retrograde) dissection/re-entry strategies when a bifurcation is present at the proximal or distal CTO cap.
c. Whenever possible, perform side-branch protection with a second guidewire.

Treatment
a. Antegrade wiring of the occluded branch (which may be challenging if dissection/re-entry strategies were used for crossing).

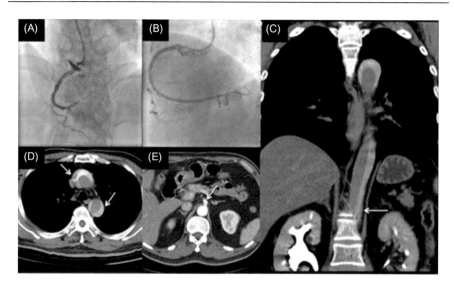

Figure 12.6 Example of aortocoronary dissection extending into the descending aorta after CTO intervention. Angiography demonstrating proximal long segment dissection of the RCA, extending to the sinus of Valsalva (A and B). After stenting with a 3.5 × 24-mm bare metal stent, the final angiogram revealed limited dissection to the sinus of Valsalva (B). Computed tomography imaging demonstrated a type A aortic dissection extending from the ascending aorta to the suprarenal abdominal level (C and D) with involvement of the aortic arch and celiac trunk (E). *Source*: Reproduced with permission from Ref. 10.

b. Retrograde recanalization of the occluded branch (if collaterals to that branch exist, Figure 5.14).
c. Use of intravascular ultrasound (IVUS) may facilitate the identification of the cause of side-branch occlusion (e.g., the presence of a subintimal track at the level of the side-branch ostium) and rewiring (Figure 12.8).

If a dissection/re-entry strategy is used, it is important to minimize the extent of the subintimal dissection by re-entering into the true lumen at the most proximal location possible: this strategy has been named limited antegrade subintimal tracking (LAST) and redirection, as described in Chapter 5.[12] Moreover, using the CrossBoss catheter may minimize the extent of subintimal dissection and facilitate re-entry attempts. The presence of a coronary bifurcation at the distal CTO cap may favor use of a primary retrograde approach to minimize the risk for side-branch occlusion during antegrade crossing attempts.

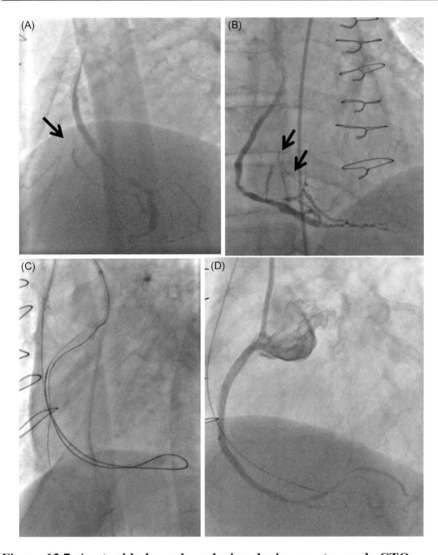

Figure 12.7 Acute side-branch occlusion during a retrograde CTO intervention. CTO of the mid RCA that filled by a diffusely diseased saphenous vein graft (A). A large acute marginal branch originated at the distal CTO cap (arrow, A and arrows, B). Successful retrograde recanalization was achieved using a retrograde true lumen puncture technique (C). Stent placement restored antegrade flow to the distal RCA but the acute marginal branch became occluded leading to inferolateral ST-segment elevation and postprocedural acute myocardial infarction. *Source*: Reproduced with permission from Ref. 11.

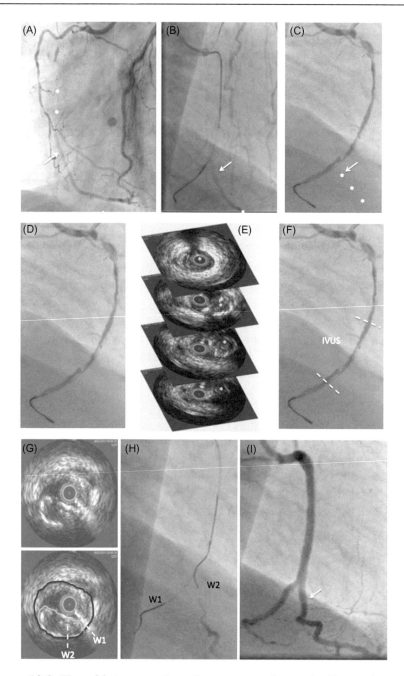

Figure 12.8 Use of intravascular ultrasonography to facilitate side-branch occlusion assessment and treatment. Antegrade PCI was planned in a first attempt to recanalize a long CTO located in the mid segment of the RCA (asterisks, A). Adequate progress was made using a parallel-wire technique with a polymer-jacketed guidewire and a blunt-tip coil wire down

12.1.1.1.4   Collateral Occlusion

Occlusion of a single large collateral (usually epicardial) vessel may cause severe ischemia and hemodynamic instability; therefore there should be a high threshold for performing retrograde CTO PCI through such collaterals. Moreover, successful CTO recanalization causes rapid "de-recruitment" of the collateral circulation, resulting in severe ischemia, if the vessel re-occludes.[13]

12.1.1.1.5   Subintimal Stenting

Occasionally, subintimal distal position of the guidewire may not be appreciated and stents may be inadvertently deployed within the subintimal space, obstructing the outflow of the vessel (Figure 12.9).[14] After this occurs, the patient may remain asymptomatic[15,16] or may develop ST-segment elevation due to side-branch loss.[14]

Causes
a. Misjudgment on the guidewire position before stent implantation, i.e., impression that the wire is located in the distal true lumen, when in reality it is located in the subintimal space.

Prevention
The first step in preventing this complication is to have a high threshold of suspicion. For example, apparent intraluminal position distal to the CTO when using a wire knuckle or very aggressive guidewires (≥ 12 gr tapered-tip wires, for example) should always raise the concern that the wire might actually be in the subintimal space close to the lumen, and be followed by an adequate check before proceeding to balloon dilation and stenting.

◄ to the posterolateral branch (B). However, antegrade injections after predilation with a 1.5-mm balloon revealed occlusion of the posterior descending artery (asterisks, C). Intravascular ultrasound of the mid RCA and crux (E and F) revealed subadventitial course of the wire located in the posterolateral artery with compression of the vessel structures at the level of the RCA crux (stars in IVUS shown in E). IVUS-guided re-entry to the posterior descending artery (PDA) with a new wire (W2) was performed (IVUS shadows of both guidewires are shown in G). This allowed successful advancement of W2 into the PDA (H) with a good result using a provisional stenting technique (I).
Source: Courtesy of Dr. Javier Escaned.

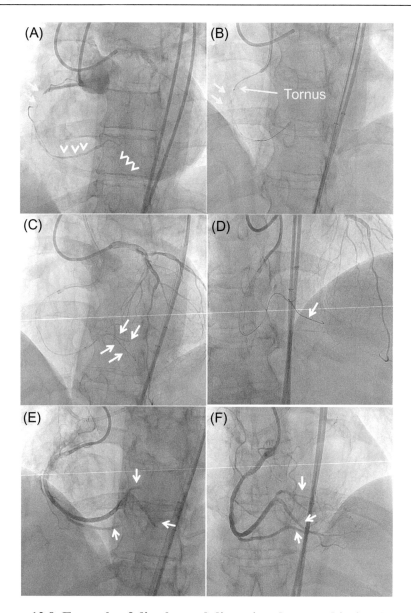

Figure 12.9 Example of distal vessel dissection due to subintimal stenting. Coronary angiography demonstrating a CTO of the mid RCA (arrows, A). The distal RCA and the right posterior descending artery (arrowheads, A) were filling via collaterals from the LAD artery. The RCA was crossed antegradely with a Pilot 200 wire, however, no other catheter,

To confirm that the wire has entered the distal true lumen *before* balloon dilation and stenting the following methods can be used:

a. **Contralateral injection**. This is the most commonly used method and is crucial for nearly all CTO procedures, even when most collaterals are ipsilateral, because ipsilateral collaterals may become compromised during crossing attempts.[17,18] After CTO crossing, it is recommended to check intraluminal position of the guidewire in two orthogonal angiographic projections.

b. **Contrast injection through a microcatheter**. Routine use of this maneuver is discouraged, since antegrade contrast injection through a microcatheter always entails the risk of subintimal space "staining" and dissection propagation if the wire is not in the distal true lumen, which can then hinder subsequent re-entry attempts. In selected cases, controlled microcatheter tip injections can be performed with care to verify intraluminal location, always checking for the "back bleeding sign" (blood coming out of the microcatheter after waiting for at least 30 s after withdrawing the guidewire).

c. **Intravascular imaging**. Intravascular ultrasound, particularly with a short-tip IVUS probe (Section 2.8) that is less likely to extend the suspected dissection, can be of great help in establishing a subintimal course.[19] Optical coherence tomography (OCT) has recently been reported as an alternative[20] but is hampered by the limited penetration of OCT imaging, the distance of the OCT lens from the catheter tip, and the need to perform contrast injections that may propagate a subintimal dissection.

d. **Observing the wire movement into distal branches**. This is suggestive of true lumen position[21] but may also be misleading as the wire can advance subintimally into side branches.

such as the Tornus catheter (arrow, B), could cross the occlusion. The RCA occlusion was crossed with a second Pilot 200 wire (arrows, C). Although contralateral injection suggested intraluminal distal wire position (arrow, D), after stenting antegrade flow in the acute marginal branch, right posterior descending artery and right posterolateral branch (arrows, E) ceased. After rewiring and balloon angioplasty of the acute marginal branch, right posterior descending artery and right posterolateral branch (arrows, F), antegrade coronary flow was restored in all three vessels. *Source*: Reproduced with permission from Future Medicine Ltd.[14]

Treatment
> If subintimal guidewire position is confirmed, re-entering the distal true lumen can be achieved using several strategies:[11]
> **a.** Stingray system.[22,23]
> **b.** Retrograde crossing of the target vessel.[18]
> **c.** Wire-based techniques, such as the subintimal tracking and re-entry (STAR) technique)[24] or preferably the LAST and mini-STAR[25] techniques, in which the area of subintimal dissection is limited by re-entering the true lumen as close as possible to the distal cap without propagating the dissection into the distal part of the vessel, as described in Chapter 5.
> **d.** IVUS-guided re-entry, following a similar technique as shown in Figure 12.8.

These same techniques can also be employed to re-enter the true lumen in cases of inadvertent diagnostic or guide catheter-induced dissection during vessel engagement or in cases of angioplasty-induced dissections followed by loss of guidewire position.[26]

12.1.1.1.6 Distal Vessel Dissection
Similar to inadvertent subintimal stenting described above, occasionally distal vessel dissection may occur, hindering further attempts to re-enter into the distal true lumen.

Causes
a. Subintimal wire crossing with failed re-entry attempts, often causing subintimal hematoma that compresses the distal true lumen.
b. Use of stiff and/or tapered-tip guidewires that may dissect the distal vessel.

Prevention
a. Avoid use of large loops during subintimal dissection techniques. It is best to perform the distal part of dissection with the CrossBoss catheter to minimize the extent of subintimal dissection.
b. Avoid antegrade contrast injections if the wire enters the subintimal space.
c. Prevent excessive movement of stiff and/or tapered-tip guidewires, for example, by using the "trapping technique" for equipment exchanges.

Treatment
a. Use the subintimal transcatheter withdrawal (STRAW) technique (as described in Figure 5.12) to aspirate the subintimal hematoma and re-expand the distal true lumen.

b. Use retrograde crossing into the distal true lumen.
c. Perform balloon angioplasty in the subintimal space and stop the procedure. Coronary angiography can be repeated after 2–3 months to allow for healing of the dissection. Occasionally, flow into the distal true lumen is restored at follow-up angiography.

12.1.1.2 Perforation

Coronary perforation is one of the most feared complications of CTO PCI, as it can lead to pericardial effusion and tamponade, sometimes necessitating emergency pericardiocentesis (and rarely cardiac surgery) to be controlled. Although coronary perforations are common in CTO PCI (27.6% in one series[27]), most perforations do not have serious consequences, and the risk of tamponade is low, approximately 0.3%.[2] In contrast to PCI of non-CTO vessels, occlusion of a perforated target vessel in CTO PCI usually does not cause myocardial ischemia, allowing for testing sequential strategies, preparing hardware, etc.

12.1.1.2.1 Perforation Classification

Coronary perforations are best classified according to location, as location has important implications regarding management. There are three main perforation locations: (i) main vessel perforation, (ii) distal artery wire perforation, and (iii) collateral vessel perforation, in either a septal or an epicardial collateral (Figure 12.10).[1]

The severity of coronary perforations has traditionally been graded using the Ellis classification:[28]

- Class 1: A crater extending outside the lumen only in the absence of linear staining angiographically suggestive of dissection.
- Class 2: Pericardial or myocardial blush without a ≥ 1-mm exit hole.
- Class 3: Frank streaming of contrast through a ≥ 1-mm exit hole.
- Class 3—cavity spilling: Perforation into an anatomic cavity chamber, such as the coronary sinus and the right ventricle.

The above classification has to be adapted to various scenarios discussed below that were not contemplated at the time the Ellis classification was developed (i.e., perforation of epicardial and septal collateral channels).

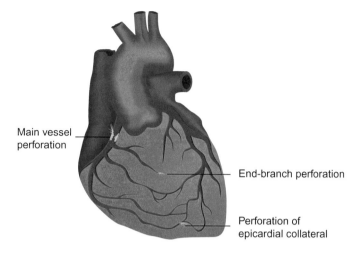

Main vessel perforation

End-branch perforation

Perforation of epicardial collateral

Figure 12.10 Illustration of the various coronary perforation types.
Source: Reproduced with permission from Ref. 1.

Prevention
1. Balloon dilation should not be performed when the guidewire is not confirmed to be within the vessel architecture.
2. In some CTOs, negative vessel remodeling may occur, facilitating vessel rupture during dilation if the balloon is sized according to proximal vessel dimensions. IVUS imaging can be of great help in clarifying the vessel size distal to the CTO.
3. Whenever a large balloon is required in CART and reverse CART procedures to facilitate guidewire passage, use of IVUS can facilitate safe balloon size selection (75% of intra-medial vessel diameter).
4. During over-the-wire device exchanges, uncontrolled advancement of a hydrophilic or polymer-jacketed wire to a distal small branch may cause distal vessel perforation. Use of balloon trapping (first choice) or wire extensions (second choice) are preferred whereas Nanto's maneuver (saline injection through the microcatheter - also called "hydraulic exchange") should be avoided.
5. Outlining the anatomy of a collateral channel before and during its crossing, either with bilateral angiography or selective tip injections with the microcatheter, can help prevent guidewire exit and channel perforation.
6. Double coil tip wires (Section 2.4.4) have excellent torque control and a blunt tip that, compared with polymer-jacketed guidewires, is less likely to cause collateral channel perforation. Hence double coil tip wires (such as the Sion wire, Asahi) should be considered as the first choice for collateral crossing.

7. In general, perforation of an epicardial collateral channel is more difficult to control than a septal one, and this fact should be taken into consideration when choosing the most adequate interventional collateral channel.
8. Unfractionated heparin is preferred for anticoagulation, as it can be reversed in case of perforation, in contrast to bivalirudin.
9. A glycoprotein IIb/IIIa inhibitor should not be administered during CTO PCI, even after successful crossing and stenting, as it may cause an unrecognized perforation to bleed.

12.1.1.2.2 General Treatment of Perforations

Treatments specific to the perforation are described in the following section. General measures that can decrease the risk of continued bleeding into the pericardium include the following:

a. **Balloon inflation** proximal to the perforation to stop the bleeding. This should be performed immediately to prevent accelerated accumulation of blood in the pericardial space and tamponade. Since a second arterial access is usually available in CTO PCI for contralateral injections, in many cases it can be used to introduce a second guide catheter with specific hardware to treat the perforation. Hemostasis at the site of perforation can be maintained with an inflated balloon through the first guide catheter.
b. **Reversal of anticoagulation** by administering protamine. Platelet administration can help reverse the effect of abciximab, but glycoprotein IIb/IIIa inhibitors should not be administered during CTO PCI. Many operators currently advocate not reversing anticoagulation, especially if the perforation is not massive and extravasation seems to be controlled with prolonged balloon inflation. Reversing the heparin carries the risk of guide catheter and/or target vessel thrombosis. Moreover, protamine may cause anaphylactic reactions in patients treated with NPH insulin in the past or with a history of fish allergy.[29]
c. Administration of **intravenous fluids and pressors**, and possibly atropine, if the patient develops bradycardia due to a vagal reaction.
d. Appropriate timing for performing **pericardiocentesis**: Hemodynamic instability requires immediate pericardiocentesis, yet smaller size pericardial effusions may be best managed conservatively, as the elevated pericardial pressure due to the entrance of blood into the pericardial space may help "tamponade the perforation site" and minimize the risk for further bleeding.
e. **Pericardiocentesis** can frequently be performed using X-ray guidance due to contrast exit into the pericardial space. Echocardiography remains

important for assessing the size of pericardial effusion and the result of pericardiocentesis and for determining whether pericardial bleeding continues. Use of an echocardiographic contrast agent can be useful for detecting ongoing bleeding into the pericardial space.[30]

f. Cardiac surgery notification: If pericardial bleeding continues in spite of percutaneous management attempts, cardiac surgery may be required to identify and control the site of bleeding.

12.1.1.2.3   Main Vessel Perforation

Causes

a. Implantation of oversized stents or high-pressure balloon inflations.

b. Wire exit from the vessel during CTO crossing attempts, followed by inadvertent advancement of equipment (such as balloons or microcatheters) into the pericardial space. Whereas wire perforation alone seldom causes blood extravasation and pericardial effusion (because it creates a very small, self-sealing hole), catheter/balloon advancement over the wire enlarges the hole, increasing the risk for blood extravasation. Occasionally the contrast extravasation may not occur until after a stent is placed over the perforated area.

Prevention

a. Avoid use of oversized stents and balloons.

b. Always confirm guidewire position within the vessel "architecture" (true lumen or subintimal space) before advancing other equipment.

Treatment

a. Inflate a balloon proximal to the perforation to stop the bleeding (Figures 12.11 and 12.12).

b. If extravasation persists in spite of anticoagulation reversal and prolonged balloon inflations, place a covered stent (Jostent Graftmaster or Graftmaster Rx, as described in Section 2.9.1), using a dual catheter technique.[31,32,33]

c. The **dual catheter technique** aims to minimize bleeding into the pericardium while preparing for covered stent delivery and deployment (Figure 12.11).[33] In this technique, a balloon is inserted through one guide catheter and inflated proximal to the perforation preventing bleeding, while a second guide catheter with the covered stent is advanced through the aorta to engage the same coronary ostium, next to the previous guiding catheter. The covered stent is advanced on a new wire through that second guiding catheter and placed just proximally to the

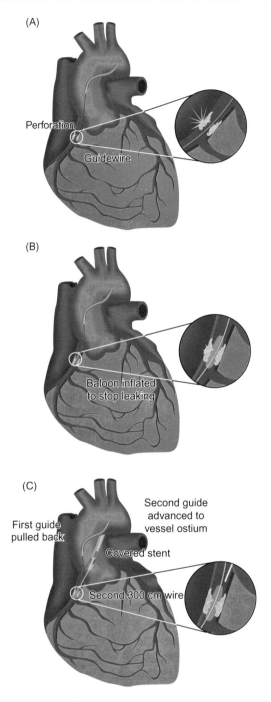

Figure 12.11 Treatment of main vessel coronary perforation. After
main vessel perforation occurs (A), a balloon is inflated at the perforation
site to stop bleeding into the pericardium (B). A second guide catheter is

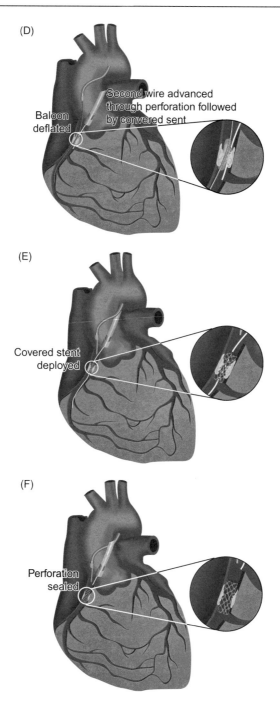

Figure 12.11 (Continued)

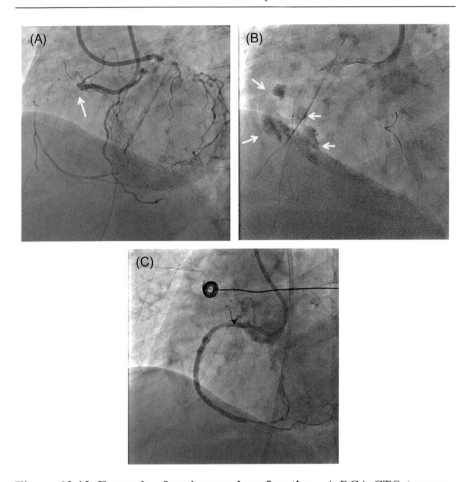

Figure 12.12 Example of main vessel perforation. A RCA CTO (arrows, A) was successfully crossed antegradely. Post-stenting angiography demonstrated a main vessel perforation with active bleeding into the pericardium (arrows, B). After implantation of a Jostent Graftmaster stent, the bleeding stopped (C).
Source: Reproduced with permission from Ref. 1.

◀ advanced to the coronary artery ostium with a covered stent over a 300-cm guidewire (C). The first guide is withdrawn and the balloon deflated, followed by wiring of the coronary artery with the second guidewire and advancement of the covered stent to the perforation site (D). Deployment of the covered stent (E) results in sealing of the perforation (F).
Source: Reproduced with permission from Ref. 1.

sealing balloon, which is briefly deflated and withdrawn proximally to allow passage of the wire and the covered stent. Use of the dual guide catheter technique minimizes the time that the perforation remains unsealed.[33]

12.1.1.2.4 Distal Wire Perforation

Distal wire perforations (Figures 12.13 and 12.14) can occasionally be difficult to diagnose, especially when collimation is used to minimize radiation exposure. Because blood flow into the pericardium may be slow, tamponade may not occur until several hours after the procedure has ended. Patients with distal wire perforation should be monitored closely and should not receive a glycoprotein IIb/IIIa inhibitor, as tamponade may not develop until hours after the end of PCI.

Causes
a. Inadvertent advancement of a guidewire and/or microcatheter into a distal small branch. Stiff, tapered, and polymer-jacketed guidewires are more likely to cause such perforations.

Prevention
Distal wire perforation can be prevented by:
a. Paying meticulous attention to distal guidewire position during attempts to deliver equipment, especially when stiff and polymer-jacketed wires are used, as those are more likely to perforate compared to workhorse guidewires.
b. Using the trapping technique to minimize wire movement during equipment exchanges.
c. Exchanging a stiff or polymer-jacketed guidewire for a workhorse guidewire immediately after confirmation of successful crossing.

Treatment
a. Prolonged proximal balloon inflation.
b. If distal wire perforation is not sealed by prolonged balloon inflation and by reversing anticoagulation, embolization of the bleeding vessel may be required using coils (see Section 2.9.2),[34] subcutaneous fat, clotted blood, thrombin,[35] or other materials (Figure 12.13).
c. Alternatively, a microcatheter may be advanced to the perforation site and suction applied, collapsing the vessel to achieve hemostasis.[36]

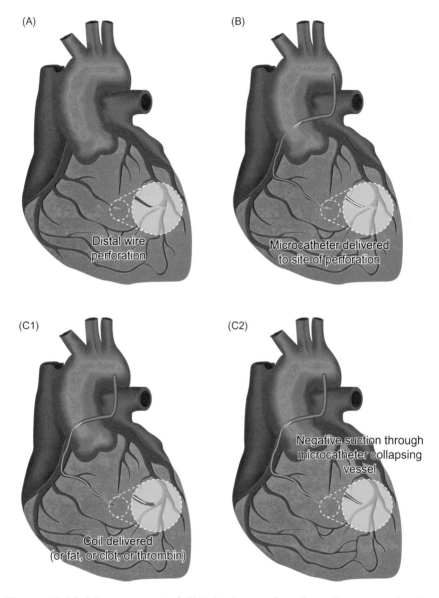

Figure 12.13 Management of distal wire perforation. To treat a distal guidewire perforation (A), a microcatheter is advanced proximal to the perforation (B) and either a coil (or other material, such as subcutaneous fat or a thrombus) is released (C1) or suction is applied through the microcatheter collapsing the vessel (C2), sealing the perforation. Large microcatheters (such as the Progreat or Transit) should be used for coil delivery, as this is not feasible through smaller microcatheters (such as the Finecross or Corsair) that are routinely used for CTO crossing.
Source: Reproduced with permission from Ref. 1.

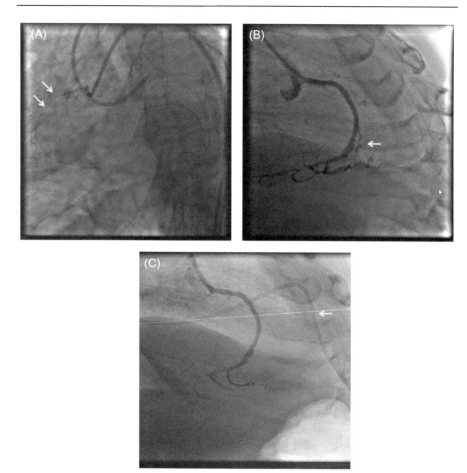

Figure 12.14 Example of distal wire perforation. An RCA CTO (arrows, A) was successfully crossed antegradely using a 12-gram-tip guidewire. Post-stenting angiography demonstrated a side-branch perforation with active bleeding into the pericardium (arrow, B). Emergency pericardiocentesis was performed (arrow, C). Delivery of a covered stent failed, but after prolonged balloon inflation and reversal of anticoagulation the side-branch bleeding stopped.
Source: Reproduced with permission from Ref. 1.

12.1.1.2.5   Collateral Vessel Perforation
Perforation of an epicardial collateral branch is a serious complication of retrograde CTO PCI, as it can rapidly lead to tamponade and may be particularly difficult to control. In contrast, perforation of

septal collaterals is unlikely to have adverse consequences,[3] although septal hematomas (Figure 12.15)[37] and even tamponade[35] have been reported following septal wire perforation.

Although prior CABG may protect from tamponade in patients in whom epicardial collateral perforation occurs, there is a reported case of epicardial collateral perforation causing localized epicardial hematoma that produced left atrial inflow and outflow obstruction, resulting in pulmonary edema and pleural effusion.[38]

Collateral vessel perforation may occur before, during, and after collateral vessel instrumentation with guidewires or devices. A meticulous technique is recommended to ensure its prevention, detection, and management.

Septal collateral perforation

Septal rupture/hematoma has been reported to occur in up to 6.9% of cases in a single series of patients treated with a retrograde approach.[39] In case reports, septal hematomas have caused asymptomatic bigeminy and severe chest pain, appear as an echo free space in the interventricular septum on transthoracic echocardiography (Figure 12.15), and resolve spontaneously.[40] Careful attention should be paid to the collateral branch course, as a collateral that appears to be septal, may in reality be epicardial. Moreover, perforation into the coronary sinus has been reported during attempts to cross a septal collateral.[41] Perforation into a cardiac chamber usually does not cause complications; however, balloon dilation or advancement of additional equipment should be avoided.

Causes
a. Aggressive septal crossing guidewire maneuvers, especially advancing the Corsair microcatheter over the guidewire after it advances to an extraluminal location.
b. Selection of a very thin or tortuous septal channel.

Prevention
a. Selection of the most adequate interventional septal channel.
b. Caution with tip injections of contrast in collateral channels if a wedged position of the microcatheter is suspected. The "back bleeding" sign observed at the hub of the microcatheter may help in preventing injections that may cause barotrauma and rupture. In the absence of this sign,

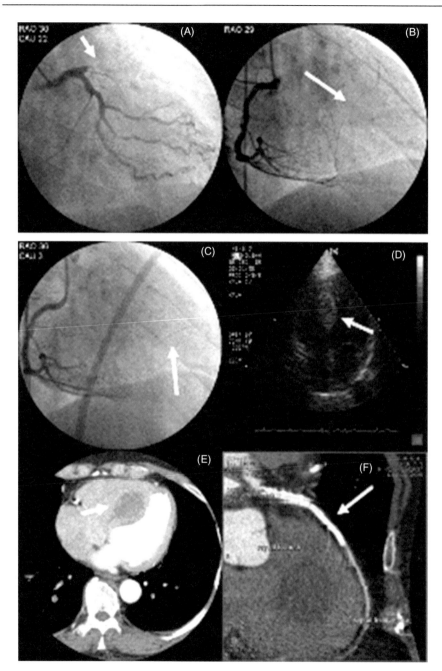

Figure 12.15 Example of septal hematoma due to septal collateral perforation. Left coronary angiography demonstrating an LAD artery CTO (arrow, A) and septal collaterals (arrow, B) from the RCA to the LAD. Retrograde wiring was attempted (arrow, C) but was unsuccessful and the CTO was recanalized using the antegrade approach. Patient developed chest

it might be worth withdrawing the microcatheter tip to a slightly more proximal location.

c. Avoiding to advance the Corsair microcatheter, until the guidewire position (within the collateral vessel or the distal true lumen) has been ascertained.

d. Withdrawal of guidewires and microcatheters from collaterals after completion of CTO recanalization should be performed after collateral perforation has been ruled out. Bilateral injection while maintaining the retrograde wire position through the collateral vessel are useful.

Treatment

a. Usually no specific treatment is required, as septal perforation are self-limiting.

b. Advancing the microcatheter is frequently enough to control bleeding.

c. Negative pressure applied from the wedged microcatheter contributes to collateral channel collapse and rupture sealing.

d. If tamponade occurs, the perforated collateral may need to be coiled.

Epicardial collateral perforation

Epicardial collateral perforation is riskier than septal collateral perforation, as it can rapidly lead to tamponade. Hence, wiring epicardial collaterals should only be performed by operators experienced in the retrograde approach. Epicardial collateral wiring is safer in patients with prior coronary bypass graft surgery or other surgery requiring opening of the pericardial sac, as bleeding may be contained within pericardial "pockets" (although tamponade can still occur[42]).

Causes

a. Aggressive guidewire advancement, especially through tortuous epicardial collaterals.

b. Advancement of microcatheters or other equipment after guidewire perforation has occurred.

◄ pain after the procedure and had increased cardiac biomarkers. Echocardiography demonstrated a mass (arrow, D) within the interventricular septum and computed tomography confirmed a septal hematoma (arrow, E) and patent stents in the LAD (arrow, F).
Source: Reproduced with permission from Ref. 37.

Prevention

a. Epicardial collaterals should be wired using a "contrast-guided" technique with selective angiography using the microcatheter (tip injections). "Surfing" should **never** be performed in epicardial collaterals.

b. In contrast to septal collaterals, epicardial collaterals should **never** be dilated. However, the septal dilator catheter (Corsair) can be used in epicardial collaterals paying careful attention to avoid catheter advancement in front of the guidewire.

Treatment

a. General perforation treatment measures should be employed, as described in Section 12.1.1.2.2.

b. In general, epicardial channel perforation is treacherous, with high risk of causing tamponade; therefore, this complication should be taken seriously, ensuring adequate correction.

c. Negative pressure applied from the wedged microcatheter can cause collateral channel collapse and rupture sealing.

d. Advancing the microcatheter is frequently enough to control bleeding through ruptured epicardial channels.

e. If tamponade occurs, the perforation may need to be embolized/coiled (Figure 12.16). Embolization should ideally be performed on both sides of the perforation, as blood flow can continue retrogradely in spite of occluding the antegrade collateral limb (Figure 12.16).

f. This may not be feasible in cases in which the CTO cannot and has not been recanalized (Figure 12.17). Although in most of such cases selective embolization of the collateral channel proximal to the perforation is sufficient to cause hemostasis (after proximal coil implantation, retrograde intra-channel pressure from an occluded vessel is low, Figure 12.18), bilateral angiography is always mandatory to rule out retrograde bleeding, which might eventually constitute an indication for cardiac surgery.

12.1.1.3 Equipment Loss or Entrapment

Equipment delivery may be challenging in CTO vessels that are frequently tortuous and calcified. Stent loss or wire entrapment may ensue.[43]

Causes

a. Attempting to deliver equipment via tortuous and calcified vessels.

b. Meeting of an antegrade balloon or stent with a retrograde Corsair catheter over the same guidewire.

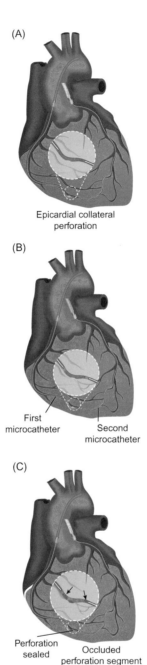

(A)

Epicardial collateral
perforation

(B)

First
microcatheter

Second
microcatheter

(C)

Perforation
sealed

Occluded
perforation segment

Figure 12.16 Management of epicardial collateral perforation. To treat
an epicardial collateral perforation (A), two microcatheters are advanced
through both the antegrade and retrograde guide catheter on both ends of
the perforation site, and a coil is released via both microcatheters (B)
sealing the perforation (C).
Source: Reproduced with permission from Ref. 1.

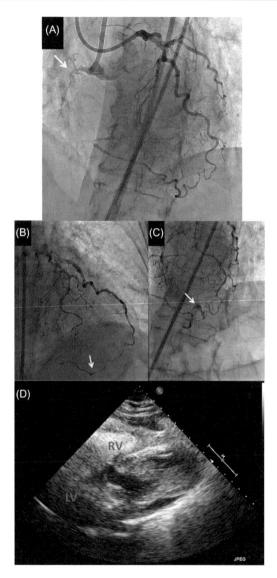

Figure 12.17 Example of epicardial collateral perforation. A retrograde
crossing attempt was performed to treat a patient with a proximal RCA
CTO (arrow, A). However, during attempts to cross the epicardial collateral
from the diagonal to the right posterior descending artery, perforation
occurred (arrow, B). After prolonged balloon inflation and reversal of
anticoagulation bleeding through the perforation stopped (arrow, C), as
confirmed by injection of echocardiographic contrast (D).
Source: Reproduced with permission from Ref. 1.

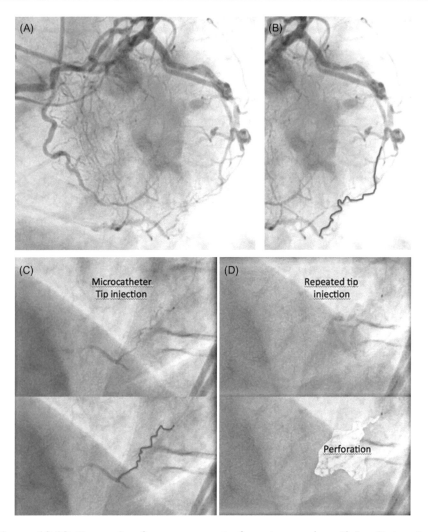

Figure 12.18 Example of management of rupture epicardial collateral channel with coil embolization. (A and B): Angiographic images obtained in a patient undergoing a second PCI attempt of a RCA CTO, several weeks after an antegrade PCI approach had failed to open the vessel. An interventional epicardial collateral with CC2 quality, connecting the circumflex artery and the posterolateral RCA branch (blue line, B), was chosen to perform retrograde PCI. Instrumentation of the collateral with a double-coil, tapered, blunt-tip wire (Sion Blue) was performed under guidance with tip injections performed through a Finecross microcatheter (C). Despite this, a perforation with fast contrast spilling was noted after

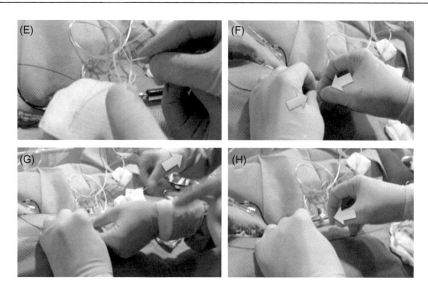

Figure 12.18 (Continued)

attempts to cross the tortuous channel (D). Negative pressure was applied to the microcatheter, without adequate hemostasis. The microcatheter was exchanged by a 0.021-in. Progreat microcatheter. An 0.018-in. Interlock coil (E) was inserted through the Progreat microcatheter while keeping tight the coil sleeve and the microcatheter hub (arrows, F). The images obtained during this PCI show how, once the coil was advanced inside the microcatheter, the sleeve was withdrawn (G), and the interlocked coil and its core wire was advanced under fluoroscopic control (F). The coil was positioned as close as possible to the perforation site (red circle), ensuring as much folding as possible of the coil (I) and eventually was released (J) (blue arrow shows how the coil is no longer locked once its junction with the core wire leaves the microcatheter tip). Complete interruption of bleeding was ensured by making simultaneous retrograde and antegrade injections (blue lines, K). Anticoagulation was not reversed during the treatment of collateral channel rupture. Antegrade PCI was then successfully performed during the same procedure (L) with implantation of a bioresorbable scaffold (Absorb) (blue arrows). The patient evolved favorably, with follow-up angiography performed 8 months later showing an excellent long-term result in the RCA.
Source: Courtesy of Dr. Javier Escaned.

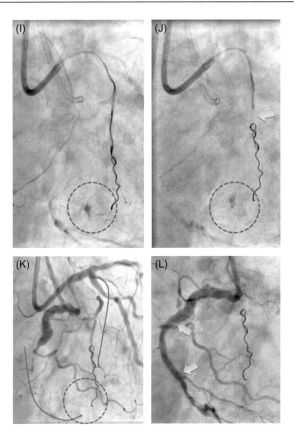

Figure 12.18 (Continued)

c. Attempting to deliver equipment via a collateral during the retrograde approach to CTO interventions (that can predispose to both stent loss[44] and wire entrapment[45]).

d. Excessive torque applied to guidewires when the tip is entrapped in the CTO or when the wire fails to transmit its torque due to wire kinking.

e. Excessive rotation applied to a Tornus microcatheter, which may cause major distortion of its structure, with high risk of device entrapment.

f. Rotation applied to wire knuckles that might cause a wire knot, making impossible its retrieval through microcatheters.

g. Aggressive advancement of a rotational atherectomy burr.

Prevention
a. Careful preparation of the CTO target vessel before stenting (with balloon angioplasty, rotational atherectomy, etc.) before attempting to deliver stents.
b. Awareness of the force applied for advancing devices when using an externalized guidewire.
c. Regularly checking that the Tornus and other microcatheters can be withdrawn before further advancement.
d. Limiting the number of turns applied to the Tornus to a maximum of 10 (either anticlockwise during advancement or clockwise during its retrieval); then releasing the device to dissipate accumulated torque.
e. Checking visually the transmission of torque to the guidewire tip. In drilling maneuvers, it is advisable to limit turns to 360°, alternating clockwise and counterclockwise rotation.
f. Never allowing the tip of an antegrade microcatheter, balloon, or stent to meet with the tip of the retrograde microcatheter over the same guidewire.
g. Whenever possible, avoiding very tortuous epicardial collateral channels that may predispose to wire entrapment.
h. First delivering more distal and then more proximal stents, as attempting to deliver a stent through an already deployed stent may cause the stent to be dislodged or lost.[43]
i. If rotational atherectomy is used, slow advancement of the burr using a pecking motion and minimizing decelerations can help ablate more tissue before the lesion is actually crossed by the burr, hence minimizing the risk of entrapment.[46,47]

Treatment
a. First, determine whether it is best to attempt retrieval of the lost equipment or deploy/crush the lost equipment. Stent deployment in a coronary segment that is unlikely to be significantly affected by stenting may be the most time-efficient and low-risk strategy, as stent retrieval attempts can prolong the procedure, increase radiation exposure, and result in distal stent embolization or target vessel injury.[43,45,48]
b. If "crushing" or deployment of the lost stent (or encasing of a guidewire fragment with stents[45]) is selected, then intravascular imaging is important to ensure that there is adequate coverage of the lost equipment and that there is no wire unraveling extending proximally in the coronary artery or even into the aorta.[43]
c. If retrieval of lost devices (usually stents) is selected, it can be accomplished using various techniques, such as the small balloon technique, and snaring (Figure 12.19).

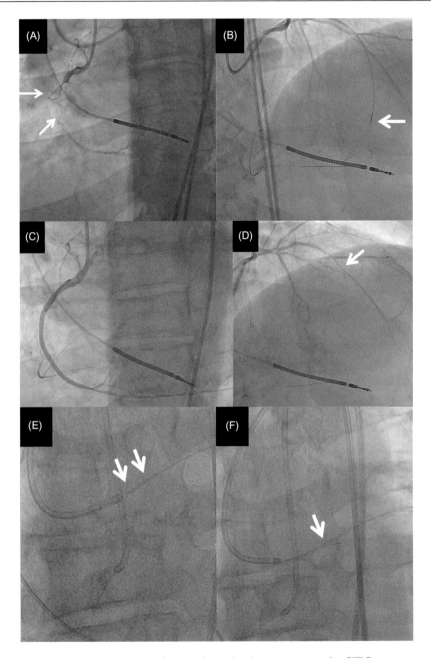

Figure 12.19 Illustration of stent loss during retrograde CTO PCI. Antegrade attempts for crossing a mid RCA CTO (arrows, A) failed due to subintimal wire passage. A Fielder FC guidewire was advanced retrogradely via a septal collateral over a Corsair catheter (arrow, B). The Corsair catheter was advanced distal to the CTO, followed by retrograde

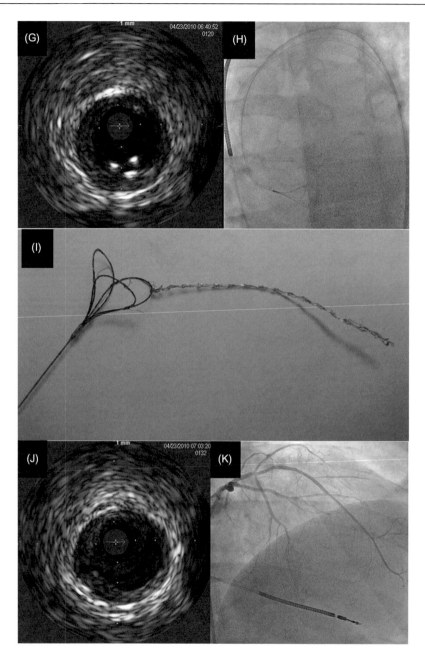

Figure 12.19 (Continued)

d. The small balloon technique can be used to retrieve a lost stent if wire position is maintained within the stent. A small balloon is advanced through the stent, inflated distal to the stent, and then withdrawn together with the lost stent into the guide catheter.

e. Various snares can be used for retrieving the lost equipment, most commonly the three-loop snares, as described in Section 2.6).

f. Advancement of several wires in parallel to an entrapped one, followed by multiple turns to "wrap" it, can be considered.

g. Controlled rupture of the wire might be considered in some cases, taking into account that frequently this leads to unfolding of the tip coil into a small filament (Figure 12.20).

h. In general, strong traction should be avoided and, if required, potential associated risks should be taken into account and minimized. For example, since left main or proximal vessel dissection may occur as a result of trauma during device traction, it is important to ensure that trapped wires are covered by a microcatheter.

i. Trapping the target device with a balloon close to the guiding catheter tip, followed by traction using the guiding catheter, should be considered; this maneuver decreases the length of the device to which traction is applied and the risk of device rupture.

If a rotational atherectomy burr becomes entrapped, a second guidewire is passed across the area of the entrapped burr and balloon inflations are performed over the second wire to "free" the burr.[46] The wire and balloon can be advanced through the same guide catheter (if 8 Fr guide catheters are used or if the Rotablator catheter is cut and the drive shaft sheath is removed), through a second guide catheter,[49] or by exchanging the original guide catheter over the Rotablator catheter shaft for a larger guide catheter.[50]

◀ true lumen puncture, as confirmed by intravascular ultrasonography. Following retrograde balloon dilation antegrade wiring was successful and after DES implantation in the RCA TIMI 3 flow was restored (C). Imaging of the LAD artery lesion revealed a lesion (arrow, D) at the site of the crossed collateral. During attempts to treat this lesion, a 2.5 × 28 mm stent was lost in the left main artery (arrows, E) and was snared by a Micro Snare Elite (arrow, F) but remained partially in the aorta and partially in the left main, as confirmed by intravascular ultrasound (G). After snaring with an En Snare (H) the stent was successfully retrieved (I), as confirmed by intravascular ultrasound (J). The LAD artery patency was restored after stenting (K).

Source: Reproduced with permission from HMP Communications.[43]

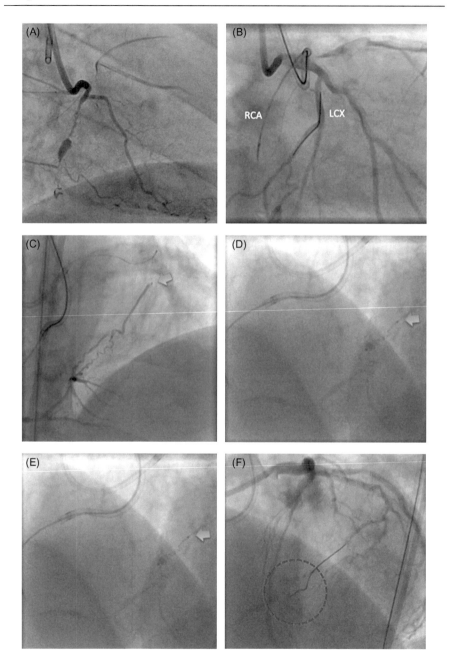

Figure 12.20 Example of wire entrapment during retrograde CTO PCI. A complex RCA CTO was approached with a combined antegrade and retrograde technique (A). Being unable to make adequate progress antegradely, a retrograde approach through CC2 epicardial channels originating in the circumflex and following a left atrial course to the posterolateral RCA branch was attempted (B). Outlining of the anatomy with tip injections performed

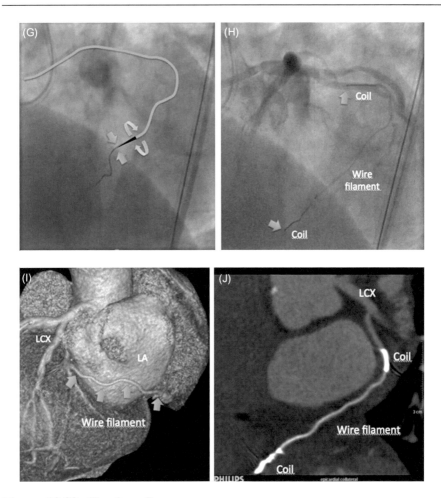

Figure 12.20 (Continued)

through a Finecross microcatheter revealed a very tortuous anatomy (C−E). A double coil, tapered blunt tip wire (Sion Blue) was advanced with caution but eventually became entrapped in the collateral channels (red circle, F). Eventually, the Finecross microcatheter was exchanged for a Corsair channel dilator, and multiple rotations of the wire and the Corsair were performed with the tip as close as possible to the location of the wire entrapment, in an attempt to perform a controlled rupture of the guidewire (G). This was achieved with two segments of the coil joined by a thin filament broken from the guidewire shaft (H). CTO revascularization was eventually not possible. Multidetector computed coronary angiography confirmed that the wire filament had not reached a major branch and no additional actions were required (I and J). *Source*: Courtesy of Dr. Javier Escaned.

12.1.2 Acute Cardiac Non-Coronary Complications

Non-coronary cardiac complications include periprocedural myocardial infarction, arrhythmias, and tamponade. Tamponade is the result of coronary perforation and has been discussed in detail in Section 12.1.1.2. Arrhythmias can complicate CTO PCI but are infrequent and are usually caused by ischemia.

Postprocedural myocardial infarction is also an infrequent complication of CTO PCI; however, its incidence is likely underdiagnosed due to lack of systematic screening with postprocedural serial cardiac troponin or CK-MB measurements.[51] Several mechanisms may lead to periprocedural myocardial injury or infarction during CTO PCI:[1]

a. Side-branch occlusion.[52]
b. Collateral vessel occlusion or injury, especially when collateral flow is provided by a single collateral (usually epicardial).
c. Injury of the target vessel distal to the CTO due to subintimal wire passage.
d. Donor vessel injury and/or thrombus and air embolization, as discussed in Section 12.1.1.

Compared to antegrade, retrograde CTO PCI may be associated with higher rates of postprocedural cardiac biomarker elevation, but its impact on acute and long-term clinical outcomes remains controversial.[51] Meticulous attention to prevent vessel occlusion and perforation and equipment loss can help minimize the risk for post-PCI myocardial infarction.

12.1.3 Other Acute General Complications

CTO interventions are subject to the same risks as non-CTO interventions.[1]

Vascular access complications can occur, especially given the frequent use of large sheaths in both femoral arteries (Section 3.4). Using unilateral or bilateral radial access[53] could potentially reduce the risk of vascular access complications but may not provide adequate backup support and limits use of the trapping technique for equipment exchanges (Section 3.7). Moreover, femoral access can provide more support for retrograde collateral channel crossing and retrograde CTO PCI. Using fluoroscopy or ultrasonography to choose the femoral arterial puncture site may reduce the risk for vascular access complications.[54,55] Routine performance of iliofemoral angiography at the time of diagnostic angiography before referral for CTO PCI can also be very useful for optimal selection of the vascular access sites.

Systemic thromboembolic complications can complicate any cardiac catheterization, including CTO PCI. Careful attention to aspiration of the guide catheters after advancement through the aorta and use of 0.065 in. guidewires may help minimize "scraping" of the aorta and reduce the risk for peripheral embolization. Moreover, careful attention to anticoagulation (which is especially important for retrograde CTO PCI given the risk for donor vessel thrombosis) can minimize the risk of catheter thrombus formation and subsequent embolization.

Non-cardiac bleeding may develop during long CTO procedures with profound anticoagulation (ACT >350 s) if a known or unknown concomitant pathology (e.g., a gastrointestinal tumor) is present. This possibility should be kept in mind if repeated vasovagal episodes occur during or after the procedure in the absence of other triggering causes.

Contrast allergic reactions may be prevented by using a premedication regimen. Such a regimen usually includes a steroid, an H1 antihistamine blocker (usually diphenhydramine), and an H2 antihistamine blocker, such as cimetidine. Adequate preprocedural hydration and limiting the volume of contrast administered (ideally the total contrast volume should be $<3.7 \times$ the creatinine clearance of the patient[56]) can help minimize the risk for **contrast nephropathy**.[57]

Finally, **radiation injury** is of particular importance to CTO PCI and is discussed in detail in Chapter 10.

12.2 Long-Term Complications

The long-term durability and outcomes of CTO PCI require further study, as most studies have only reported acute procedural results.

Similar to non-CTO interventions, patients who undergo CTO PCI may subsequently experience in-stent restenosis or stent thrombosis.

The incidence of **in-stent restenosis** and the need for repeat revascularization has decreased with drug-eluting stents (DES), especially second generation DES, as described in Chapter 11. It is important to avoid stent undersizing, as the target vessel is frequently underexpanded due to chronic hypoperfusion and increases in diameter over time.

Similarly, the risk of **stent thrombosis** post-CTO stenting has received limited study but appears to be lower with second versus first generation DES, as described in Chapter 11. Use of multiple and undersized stents in CTO PCI may predispose to stent thrombosis. To minimize this risk many operators routinely administer >12 months of dual antiplatelet therapy in patients who undergo successful CTO PCI, although the safety and efficacy of this regimen in this high-risk patient group remains unknown.

Late **coronary artery aneurysm** formation may also complicate CTO PCI (Figures 12.21 and 12.22). Coronary artery aneurysms were seen in 7.3% of patients in whom retrograde intervention was performed versus 2.6% of patients in whom antegrade intervention was performed among 560 patients undergoing CTO PCI in Japan.[58] Treatment of such aneurysms is controversial due to lack of natural history data. At present a reasonable approach is to continue dual antiplatelet therapy and perform serial angiographic and intravascular imaging (with intravascular ultrasonography or ideally with OCT that has higher resolution), with aneurysm sealing limited to patients with large aneurysms or aneurysms that enlarge during follow-up.[59] Some aneurysms may spontaneously resolve during follow-up (Figure 12.22).

12.3   Conclusion

Every interventional procedure, including CTO PCI, is a balancing act between potential risks and benefits. For patients in whom successful CTO PCI can provide significant benefit, the fear of

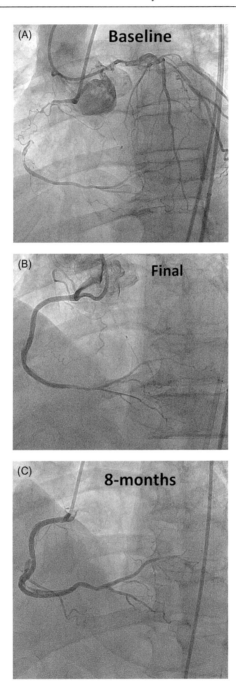

Figure 12.21 Late coronary artery aneurysm formation after CTO intervention. A RCA CTO was successfully crossed using a dissection/

(D)

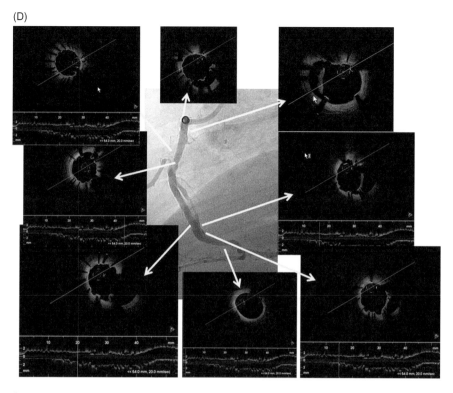

Figure 12.21 (Continued)

complications should not prevent us from performing the procedure. It should, however, prompt us to meticulously and painstakingly prepare to prevent complications and to promptly and efficiently treat them, should they occur. Our patients deserve no less.[60]

re-entry strategy and stented with three DES (B). Repeat angiography performed 8 months later revealed a mid RCA aneurysm (C), as confirmed by OCT (D). The patient remained asymptomatic and repeat coronary angiography and long-term dual antiplatelet therapy was recommended. *Source*: Reproduced with permission from Ref. 1.

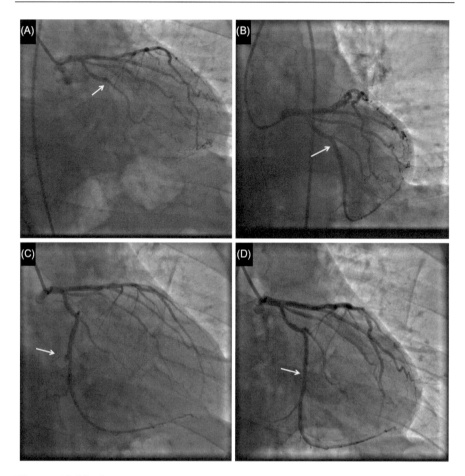

Figure 12.22 Spontaneous aneurysm resolution after CTO intervention. PCI of a mid circumflex CTO (arrow, A) was successful (arrow, B) using an antegrade dissection/re-entry technique. Follow-up angiography 3 months later demonstrated an aneurysm at the site of re-entry (arrow, C) that resolved by 10 months' post-PCI (D).
Source: Courtesy of Dr. Michael Luna.

References

1. Brilakis ES, Karmpaliotis D, Patel V, Banerjee S. Complications of chronic total occlusion angioplasty. *Interv Cardiol Clinics* 2012;**1**:373−89.
2. Patel VG, Brayton KM, Tamayo A, et al. Angiographic success and procedural complications in patients undergoing percutaneous coronary chronic total occlusion interventions: a weighted meta-analysis of 18,061 patients from 65 studies. *JACC Cardiovasc Interv* 2013;**6**:128−36.

3. Lee NH, Seo HS, Choi JH, Suh J, Cho YH. Recanalization strategy of retrograde angioplasty in patients with coronary chronic total occlusion —analysis of 24 cases, focusing on technical aspects and complications. *Int J Cardiol* 2010;**144**:219–29.

4. Ge JB, Zhang F, Ge L, Qian JY, Wang H. Wire trapping technique combined with retrograde approach for recanalization of chronic total occlusion. *Chin Med J (Engl)* 2008;**121**:1753–6.

5. Lichtenwalter C, Banerjee S, Brilakis ES. Dual guide catheter technique for treating native coronary artery lesions through tortuous internal mammary grafts: separating equipment delivery from target lesion visualization. *J Invasive Cardiol* 2010;**22**:E78–81.

6. Papayannis A, Banerjee S, Brilakis ES. Use of the CrossBoss catheter in coronary chronic total occlusion due to in-stent restenosis. *Catheter Cardiovasc Interv* 2012;**80**:E30–6.

7. Carstensen S, Ward MR. Iatrogenic aortocoronary dissection: the case for immediate aortoostial stenting. *Heart Lung Circ* 2008;**17**:325–9.

8. Gomez-Moreno S, Sabate M, Jimenez-Quevedo P, et al. Iatrogenic dissection of the ascending aorta following heart catheterisation: incidence, management and outcome. *EuroIntervention* 2006;**2**: 197–202.

9. Abdou SM, Wu CJ. Treatment of aortocoronary dissection complicating anomalous origin right coronary artery and chronic total intervention with intravascular ultrasound guided stenting. *Catheter Cardiovasc Interv* 2011;**78**:914–9.

10. Liao MT, Liu SC, Lee JK, Chiang FT, Wu CK. Aortocoronary dissection with extension to the suprarenal abdominal aorta: a rare complication after percutaneous coronary intervention. *JACC Cardiovasc Interv* 2012;**5**:1292–3.

11. Michael TT, Papayannis AC, Banerjee S, Brilakis ES. Subintimal dissection/reentry strategies in coronary chronic total occlusion interventions. *Circ Cardiovasc Interv* 2012;**5**:729–38.

12. Lombardi WL. Retrograde PCI: what will they think of next? *J Invasive Cardiol* 2009;**21**:543.

13. Zimarino M, Ausiello A, Contegiacomo G, et al. Rapid decline of collateral circulation increases susceptibility to myocardial ischemia: the trade-off of successful percutaneous recanalization of chronic total occlusions. *J Am Coll Cardiol* 2006;**48**:59–65.

14. Patel VG, Banerjee S, Brilakis ES. Treatment of inadvertent subintimal stenting during intervention of a coronary chronic total occlusion. *Interv Cardiol* 2013;**5**:165–9.

15. Omurlu K, Ozeke O. Side-by-side false and true lumen stenting for recanalization of the chronically occluded right coronary artery. *Heart Vessels* 2008;**23**:282–5.

16. Krivonyak GS, Warren SG. Compression of a subintimal or false lumen stent by stenting in the true lumen. *J Invasive Cardiol* 2001;**13**:698—701.
17. Singh M, Bell MR, Berger PB, Holmes Jr. DR. Utility of bilateral coronary injections during complex coronary angioplasty. *J Invasive Cardiol* 1999;**11**:70—4.
18. Brilakis ES, Grantham JA, Rinfret S, et al. A percutaneous treatment algorithm for crossing coronary chronic total occlusions. *JACC Cardiovasc Interv* 2012;**5**:367—79.
19. Banerjee S, Master R, Brilakis ES. Intravascular ultrasound-guided true lumen re-entry for successful recanalization of chronic total occlusions. *J Invasive Cardiol* 2010;**22**:608—10.
20. Schultz C, van der Ent M, Serruys PW, Regar E. Optical coherence tomography to guide treatment of chronic occlusions? *J Am Coll Cardiol Intv* 2009;**2**:366—7.
21. Hussain F. Distal side branch entry technique to accomplish recanalization of a complex and heavily calcified chronic total occlusion. *J Invasive Cardiol* 2007;**19**:E340—2.
22. Werner GS. The BridgePoint devices to facilitate recanalization of chronic total coronary occlusions through controlled subintimal reentry. *Expert Rev Med Devices* 2011;**8**:23—9.
23. Brilakis ES, Badhey N, Banerjee S. "Bilateral knuckle" technique and Stingray re-entry system for retrograde chronic total occlusion intervention. *J Invasive Cardiol* 2011;**23**:E37—9.
24. Colombo A, Mikhail GW, Michev I, et al. Treating chronic total occlusions using subintimal tracking and reentry: the STAR technique. *Catheter Cardiovasc Interv* 2005;**64**:407—11 [discussion 12].
25. Galassi AR, Tomasello SD, Costanzo L, et al. Mini-STAR as bail-out strategy for percutaneous coronary intervention of chronic total occlusion. *Catheter Cardiovasc Interv* 2012;**79**:30—40.
26. Martinez-Rumayor AA, Banerjee S, Brilakis ES. Knuckle wire and stingray balloon for recrossing a coronary dissection after loss of guidewire position. *JACC Cardiovasc Interv* 2012;**5**:e31—2.
27. Rathore S, Matsuo H, Terashima M, et al. Procedural and in-hospital outcomes after percutaneous coronary intervention for chronic total occlusions of coronary arteries 2002 to 2008: impact of novel guidewire techniques. *JACC Cardiovasc Interv* 2009;**2**:489—97.
28. Ellis SG, Ajluni S, Arnold AZ, et al. Increased coronary perforation in the new device era. Incidence, classification, management, and outcome. *Circulation* 1994;**90**:2725—30.

29. Stewart WJ, McSweeney SM, Kellett MA, Faxon DP, Ryan TJ. Increased risk of severe protamine reactions in NPH insulin-dependent diabetics undergoing cardiac catheterization. *Circulation* 1984;**70**:788—92.

30. Bagur R, Bernier M, Kandzari DE, Karmpaliotis D, Lembo NJ, Rinfret S. A novel application of contrast echocardiography to exclude active coronary perforation bleeding in patients with pericardial effusion. *Catheter Cardiovasc Interv* 2013;**82**:221—9.

31. Briguori C, Nishida T, Anzuini A, Di Mario C, Grube E, Colombo A. Emergency polytetrafluoroethylene-covered stent implantation to treat coronary ruptures. *Circulation* 2000;**102**:3028—31.

32. Romaguera R, Waksman R. Covered stents for coronary perforations: is there enough evidence? *Catheter Cardiovasc Interv* 2011;**78**:246—53.

33. Ben-Gal Y, Weisz G, Collins MB, et al. Dual catheter technique for the treatment of severe coronary artery perforations. *Catheter Cardiovasc Interv* 2010;**75**:708—12.

34. Rathore S, Katoh O, Matsuo H, et al. Retrograde percutaneous recanalization of chronic total occlusion of the coronary arteries: procedural outcomes and predictors of success in contemporary practice. *Circ Cardiovasc Interv* 2009;**2**:124—32.

35. Matsumi J, Adachi K, Saito S. A unique complication of the retrograde approach in angioplasty for chronic total occlusion of the coronary artery. *Catheter Cardiovasc Interv* 2008;**72**:371—8.

36. Yasuoka Y, Sasaki T. Successful collapse vessel treatment with a syringe for thrombus-aspiration after the guidewire-induced coronary artery perforation. *Cardiovasc Revasc Med* 2010;**11**(263):e1—3.

37. Lin TH, Wu DK, Su HM, et al. Septum hematoma: a complication of retrograde wiring in chronic total occlusion. *Int J Cardiol* 2006;**113**:e64—6.

38. Aggarwal C, Varghese J, Uretsky BF. Left atrial inflow and outflow obstruction as a complication of retrograde approach for chronic total occlusion: report of a case and literature review of left atrial hematoma after percutaneous coronary intervention. *Catheter Cardiovasc Interv* 2012;**82**:770—5.

39. Sianos G, Barlis P, Di Mario C, et al. European experience with the retrograde approach for the recanalisation of coronary artery chronic total occlusions. A report on behalf of the euroCTO club. *EuroIntervention* 2008;**4**:84—92.

40. Fairley SL, Donnelly PM, Hanratty CG, Walsh SJ. Images in cardiovascular medicine. Interventricular septal hematoma and ventricular septal defect after retrograde intervention for a chronic total occlusion of a left anterior descending coronary artery. *Circulation* 2010;**122**:e518—21.

41. Sachdeva R, Hughes B, Uretsky BF. Retrograde approach to a totally occluded right coronary artery via a septal perforator artery: the tale of a long and winding wire. *J Invasive Cardiol* 2010;**22**:E65−6.
42. Marmagkiolis K, Brilakis ES, Hakeem A, Cilingiroglu M, Bilodeau L. Saphenous vein graft perforation during percutaneous coronary intervention: a case series. *J Invasive Cardiol* 2013;**25**:157−61.
43. Iturbe JM, Abdel-Karim AR, Papayannis A, et al. Frequency, treatment, and consequences of device loss and entrapment in contemporary percutaneous coronary interventions. *J Invasive Cardiol* 2012;**24**: 215−21.
44. Utsunomiya M, Kobayashi T, Nakamura S. Case of dislodged stent lost in septal channel during stent delivery in complex chronic total occlusion of right coronary artery. *J Invasive Cardiol* 2009;**21**:E229−33.
45. Sianos G, Papafaklis MI. Septal wire entrapment during recanalisation of a chronic total occlusion with the retrograde approach. *Hellenic J Cardiol* 2011;**52**:79−83.
46. Rangan BV, Brilakis ES. Getting out of jail: creative solutions in a moment of crisis. *Catheter Cardiovasc Interv* 2011;**78**:571−2.
47. Kaneda H, Saito S, Hosokawa G, Tanaka S, Hiroe Y. Trapped Rotablator: kokesi phenomenon. *Catheter Cardiovasc Interv* 2000;**49**: 82−4 [discussion 5].
48. Brilakis ES, Best PJ, Elesber AA, et al. Incidence, retrieval methods, and outcomes of stent loss during percutaneous coronary intervention: a large single-center experience. *Catheter Cardiovasc Interv* 2005;**66**:333−40.
49. Grise MA, Yeager MJ, Teirstein PS. A case of an entrapped rotational atherectomy burr. *Catheter Cardiovasc Interv* 2002;**57**:31−3.
50. Hyogo M, Inoue N, Nakamura R, et al. Usefulness of conquest guidewire for retrieval of an entrapped rotablator burr. *Catheter Cardiovasc Interv* 2004;**63**:469−72.
51. Lo N, Michael TT, Moin D, et al. Periprocedural myocardial injury in chronic total occlusion percutaneous interventions: a systematic cardiac biomarker evaluation study. *JACC Cardiovasc Interv* 2013. [published online before print].
52. Paizis I, Manginas A, Voudris V, Pavlides G, Spargias K, Cokkinos DV. Percutaneous coronary intervention for chronic total occlusions: the role of side-branch obstruction. *EuroIntervention* 2009;**4**:600−6.
53. Rinfret S, Joyal D, Nguyen CM, et al. Retrograde recanalization of chronic total occlusions from the transradial approach; early Canadian experience. *Catheter Cardiovasc Interv* 2011;**78**:366−74.

54. Seto AH, Abu-Fadel MS, Sparling JM, et al. Real-time ultrasound guidance facilitates femoral arterial access and reduces vascular complications: FAUST (Femoral Arterial Access With Ultrasound Trial). *JACC Cardiovasc Interv* 2010;**3**:751−8.

55. Abu-Fadel MS, Sparling JM, Zacharias SJ, et al. Fluoroscopy vs. traditional guided femoral arterial access and the use of closure devices: a randomized controlled trial. *Catheter Cardiovasc Interv* 2009;**74**: 533−9.

56. Laskey WK, Jenkins C, Selzer F, et al. Volume-to-creatinine clearance ratio: a pharmacokinetically based risk factor for prediction of early creatinine increase after percutaneous coronary intervention. *J Am Coll Cardiol* 2007;**50**:584−90.

57. Levine GN, Bates ER, Blankenship JC, et al. 2011 ACCF/AHA/SCAI Guideline for Percutaneous Coronary Intervention: executive summary: a report of the American College of Cardiology Foundation/American Heart Association Task Force on Practice Guidelines and the Society for Cardiovascular Angiography and Interventions. *Catheter Cardiovasc Interv* 2012;**79**:453−95.

58. Tanaka H, Kadota K, Hosogi S, Fuku Y, Goto T, Mitsudo K. Mid-term angiographic and clinical outcomes from antegrade versus retrograde recanalization for chronic total occlusions. *J Am Coll Cardiol* 2011;**57**: E1628.

59. Brilakis ES, Banerjee S. Advances in the treatment of coronary artery aneurysms. *Catheter Cardiovasc Interv* 2011;**77**:1042−4.

60. Brilakis ES. Should the fear of complications stop you from doing CTO interventions? *Cardiol Today's Interv* 2013. July August 2013.

13 How to Build a Successful CTO Program

Building a successful chronic total occlusion (CTO) intervention program is best achieved using a multifaceted approach, addressing four areas: (1) CTO operator; (2) catheterization laboratory staff, equipment, and policies; (3) administration; and (4) referring physicians and patients.[1]

1. **Operator**

    The following steps can assist an interventionalist to evolve into a successful CTO operator:

    a. Reading CTO-related literature (all interventional journals; Catheterization and Cardiovascular Interventions, Journal of Invasive Cardiology, and JACC Cardiovascular Interventions provide more detailed articles on the technical and clinical aspects of CTO PCI).

    b. Participating in online CTO-related education: www.ctofundamentals. org is an outstanding website providing basic to advanced CTO PCI education; it also provides an online physician community that regularly shares cases and expertise. In some cases, success may hinge on a nuance of technique that an operator may have never done before and only be aware of through a course, www.ctofundamentals.org, or the literature.

    c. Observing CTO interventions at experienced CTO PCI centers.

    d. Attending CTO PCI courses and meetings.

    e. Getting proctored by experienced CTO interventionalists: On-the-job training is invaluable for learning CTO PCI techniques.

    f. Practicing: As with any procedure, the more CTO interventions one does, the better CTO operator he or she becomes!

    g. Working with another interventionalist during CTO PCI, if feasible, allows for real-time feedback and adaptation of the procedural plan.

    h. Meticulous procedural planning: Understanding the CTO anatomy and the possible crossing strategies facilitates efficient and confident conversion within the "hybrid" algorithm (Chapter 7).

Manual of Coronary Chronic Total Occlusion Interventions. DOI: http://dx.doi.org/10.1016/B978-0-12-420129-3.00013-1

    i. Carefully selecting patients who are likely to benefit from CTO PCI, as outlined in Chapter 1.

    j. Focusing on and practicing the basics of CTO PCI, as outlined in Chapter 3.

    k. Persisting: Committing time and energy is required for CTO PCI. Per Dr. Bill Lombardi, one of fathers of CTO interventions in North America, "you either do CTO PCI, or you don't—there is no such thing as trying." In other words, some CTO interventions can be challenging and demanding, but the key to success is persistence. With increasing experience the procedures become faster and success rates increase.[2]

    l. Being creative: Every CTO is unique and may require a different, tailored treatment approach (although an overall standardization of CTO PCI techniques, referred to as the "hybrid approach," was recently developed, as described in Chapter 7[3]).

    m. Learning from failures: Unlike non-CTO interventions, CTO PCI failure is not uncommon, especially early in the learning curve. Failed procedures should not be a source of discouragement but should rather stimulate constructive evaluation and learning. Discussing failed cases with other operators can be fruitful.

    n. Keeping track of procedural outcomes, for example, by creating a local CTO PCI database or by joining the Progress CTO PCI registry (if you are interested please contact the author at esbrilakis@gmail.com).

    o. Publishing challenging or unique CTO PCI cases, or the overall outcomes of the CTO PCI program.

2. Catheterization laboratory staff, equipment, and policies

    The importance of building a CTO team, procuring the necessary equipment, and implementing appropriate policies cannot be overemphasized, and consists of:

a. Staff education, including:
- Lectures for catheterization laboratory staff on the indications and complexity of CTO PCI.
- Identifying specific catheterization laboratory personnel "champions" who are:
  - Interested in developing further expertise in CTO PCI.
  - Interested in routinely being involved in CTO cases.

b. Obtaining the necessary equipment (Table 2.1).

c. Establishing CTO-specific protocols for:
- Radiation management (as described in detail in Chapter 10):
  - Utilizing 7.5 fps fluoroscopy.
  - Continuously monitoring radiation dose.

- Stopping the procedure if crossing has not been achieved after 7–10 Gy air kerma dose.
- Following up patients who receive >5 Gy air kerma dose to detect any skin injury.
  - Anticoagulation:
    - Repeating ACT every 30 min.
    - Goal ACT >300 s for antegrade cases.
    - Goal ACT >350 s for retrograde cases.

d. Establishing "CTO days," which allows uninterrupted and concentrated focus on CTO PCI procedures: It is important for the operator to know that he or she has no other commitments for several hours, so prolonged treatment attempts are feasible, if necessary. Moreover, dedicated "CTO days" can improve staff acceptance of starting a CTO program, facilitate visits by proctors or clinical specialists, and also allow referring cardiologists to visit.

3. **Administration**

The following steps can assist with securing support from administration in order to build a CTO PCI program:

a. Highlighting the need for such a program, by showing the number of patients who could benefit from CTO PCI.

b. Demonstrating to administration that CTO PCI is both feasible and not a "money-losing" proposition. Pilot economic analyses from the Piedmont Heart Institute demonstrate similar contribution margins for CTO and non-CTO PCI.[1]

c. Highlighting the institutional benefits of a CTO PCI program (halo effect):
  - Developing regional and/or national reputation for doing complex interventions.
  - Increasing internal procedural volume.
  - Increasing outside referrals.

4. **Referring physicians and patients**

Increasing the awareness of the CTO PCI program can increase referrals of patients who may benefit from these procedures and can be accomplished by:

a. Educating referring physicians (both cardiologists and general practitioners). It is imperative for referring physicians to understand the rationale and potential clinical benefits of CTO PCI.

b. Presenting CTO PCI cases at case conferences, Grand Rounds, and Roundtables. These presentations can illustrate that many of the previously considered "undoable" procedures are actually feasible and can provide significant benefit to the patients.

c. Educating the patients. Many patients with severe angina are very motivated to find treatment options themselves. Online posting of patient brochures focusing on CTO intervention, as well as video testimonials (with appropriate patient consent) can be powerful educational tools.

In order for a CTO program to be successful, proper education of staff, administration, and referring physicians is essential. When their support is combined with the correct toolbox and operator skillset, one can develop a high-level program to offer an excellent therapeutic option to an undertreated patient population.

References

1. Karmpaliotis D, Lembo N, Kalynych A, et al. Development of a high-volume, multiple-operator program for percutaneous chronic total coronary occlusion revascularization: procedural, clinical, and cost-utilization outcomes. *Catheter Cardiovasc Interv* 2013;**82**:1−8.
2. Brilakis ES. The why and how of CTO interventions. *Cardiol Today's Interv* 2012. January/February.
3. Brilakis ES, Grantham JA, Rinfret S, et al. A percutaneous treatment algorithm for crossing coronary chronic total occlusions. *JACC Cardiovasc Interv* 2012;**5**:367−79.

Appendix 1: Equipment Commonly Utilized in CTO Interventions

Name	Type	Manufacturer	Pages
Amplatz gooseneck snare	Snare	Covidien	39
Angiosculpt	Balloon (for scoring lesions)	Angioscore	45, 46
Atrieve	Snare (3 loop)	Angiotech	39
Azur	Coil	Terumo	
Choice PT floppy	Guidewire (polymer-jacketed)	Boston Scientific	29
Corsair	Microcatheter—channel dilator	Asahi Intecc	22
Cross-it 100XT	Guidewire	Abbott Vascular	29
Crosswire NT	Guidewire	Terumo	29
Eagle Eye	Intravascular ultrasound catheter	Volcano	45
Ensnare	Snare (3 loop)	Merit Medical	39
Confianza	Guidewire (with tapered tip)	Asahi Intecc	28, 31
Confianza Pro 12	Guidewire (with tapered tip and hydrophilic coating)	Asahi Intecc	28
Co-Pilot	Y-connector with hemostatic valve	Abbott Vascular	20
CrossBoss	Microcatheter for crossing	Boston Scientific	37, 38, 100
Crusade	Dual lumen microcatheter	Kaneka Medix Corporation	81
Eaucath	Sheathless guide system	Asahi Intecc	17
Fielder FC	Guidewire (polymer-jacketed)	Asahi Intecc	28
Fielder XT	Guidewire (polymer-jacketed with tapered tip)	Asahi Intecc	28

(*Continued*)

(Continued)

Name	Type	Manufacturer	Pages
Finecross	Microcatheter	Terumo	20, 24
Gopher	Microcatheter (for "balloon uncrossable" lesions)	Vascular Solutions	
Graftmaster Rx	Covered stent (rapid-exchange)	Abbott Vascular	47, 48
Guardian	Y-connector with hemostatic valve	Vascular Solutions	16, 20
Guideliner	Guide catheter extension	Vascular Solutions	8, 43
Guidezilla	Guide catheter extension	Boston Scientific	43, 66
Interlock	Coil	Boston Scientific	49
Jostent Graftmaster	Covered stent (over-the-wire system)	Abbott Vascular	47
Minnie	Microcatheter	Vascular Solutions	21
MiracleBros 3, 4.5, 6, 12	Guidewire	Asahi Intecc	30
Pegasus	Magnetic navigation guidewire	Stereotaxis, St. Louis, Missouri	126
Persuader 3, 6, 9	Guidewire	Medtronic	30
ProVia 3, 6, 9	Guidewire	Medtronic	30
Pilot 50, 150, 200	Guidewire (polymer-jacketed)	Abbott Vascular	28, 29, 94, 108
Progreat	Microcatheter (large one— usually used for coil delivery)	Terumo	21, 24
Progress 40, 80, 120, 140T, 200T	Guidewire	Abbott Vascular	30
Prowler	Microcatheter	Cordis	21, 122
PT2 Moderate Support	Guidewire (polymer-jacketed)	Boston Scientific	29
			29

(*Continued*)

(Continued)

Name	Type	Manufacturer	Pages
PT Graphix Intermediate	Guidewire (polymer-jacketed)	Boston Scientific	
Quick-Access Needle Holder	Needle holder	Spectranetics	183, 184
Quick Cross	Microcatheter	Spectranetics	21
R350	Guidewire (for externalization)	Vascular Solutions	28, 35, 140
RadPad	Radiation shield	Worldwide Innovations & Technologies	48, 185
Renegade	Microcatheter (large one—usually used for coil delivery)	Boston Scientific	24, 48
RG3	Guidewire (for externalization)	Asahi Intecc	30, 35
Rotablator	Rotational atherectomy system	Boston Scientific	224
Rotaglide	Lubricant solution for rotational atherectomy and for wire externalization	Boston Scientific	17, 138
RotaWire Floppy and Extra support	Guidewire (for rotational atherectomy)	Boston Scientific	30
Runthrough	Guidewire (workhorse)	Terumo	29
Shinobi and Shinobi Plus	Guidewire	Cordis	29
Sion	Guidewire (first choice for collateral crossing in the retrograde approach)	Asahi Intecc	16, 35
Stingray balloon 103–104	Balloon (for re-entry into true lumen)	Boston Scientific	37, 38,

(Continued)

(Continued)

Name	Type	Manufacturer	Pages
Stingray wire	Guidewire (for re-entry through Stingray balloon)	Boston Scientific	104, 106
Supercross	Microcatheter (with angled tip)	Vascular Solutions	21, 122
Tegaderm	Sterile cover	3M	18
Titan	Magnetic navigation guidewire	Stereotaxis, St. Louis, Missouri	126
Tornus	Microcatheter (for "balloon uncrossable" lesions)	Asahi Intecc	15, 21, 41
Tracker Excel 14	Microcatheter	Boston Scientific	21
Transit	Microcatheter (large one— usually used for coil delivery)	Cordis	21, 24
Twin Pass 5200	Microcatheter (dual lumen)	Vascular Solutions	21
Valet	Microcatheter	Volcano	16, 20, 21, 24, 27
Venture	Microcatheter (with torquable distal tip)	Vascular Solutions	20, 24
Viper	Guidewire for externalization	CSI	18, 28, 35, 140
Whisper LS, MS, ES	Guidewire (polymer-jacketed)	Abbott Vascular	29

Manufacturer	Location
Abbott Vascular	Santa Clara, CA
Angioscore	Fremont, CA
Angiotech	Vancouver, BC, Canada
Asahi Intecc	Nagoya, Japan
Boston Scientific	Natick, MA
Cordis	Warren, NJ

(Continued)

Manufacturer	Location
Covidien	Plymouth, MN
CSI (Cardiovascular Systems Inc)	St Paul, MN
Medtronic	Santa Rosa, CA
Merit Medical	South Jordan, UT
Spectranetics	Colorado Springs, CO
Terumo	Somerset, NJ
Vascular Solutions	Minneapolis, MN
Volcano	San Diego, CA
Worldwide Innovations & Technologies	Kansas City, KS
3M	St Paul, MN

Appendix 2: Commonly Used Acronyms in CTO Interventions

Acronym	Full Name	Description	Page (Main Explanation)	Pages (Mentioned)
CART	Controlled antegrade and retrograde tracking and dissection	Technique for re-entry into the true lumen after subintimal CTO crossing during the retrograde approach: a balloon is inflated over the retrograde guidewire creating a space into which an antegrade guidewire is advanced.	131–133	44, 45, 49, 50, 131, 137, 144, 156, 203, 210
Confluent balloon technique	Confluent balloon technique	Variation of the CART technique in which an antegrade and a retrograde balloon are inflated simultaneously	134	131, 136

(Continued)

(Continued)

Acronym	Full Name	Description	Page (Main Explanation)	Pages (Mentioned)
		in a kissing fashion to cause the subintimal space to become confluent, allowing wire passage through the CTO.		
Contrast-guided STAR	Contrast-guided subintimal tracking and re-entry	Variation of the STAR technique introduced by Mauro Carlino in which subintimal contrast injection through a microcatheter inserted into the proximal cap is used to create/visualize a dissection plane and guide guidewire advancement.	93	94, 97, 110
IVUS-guided CART	Intravascular ultrasound-guided controlled	Variation of the reverse CART technique: IVUS is used	134, 135	131

(Continued)

Acronym	Full Name	Description	Page (Main Explanation)	Pages (Mentioned)
	antegrade and retrograde tracking and dissection	to allow more precise sizing of the balloon (to maximize the space created for re-entry without risking vessel rupture) and to determine whether significant recoil occurs after ballooning.		
LAST	Limited antegrade subintimal tracking	Wire-based antegrade dissection/re-entry technique: the CTO is crossed using a knuckle wire, followed by re-entry into the distal true lumen immediately distal to the distal cap usually using a stiff guidewire with a 90° bend —this is in contrast to the STAR technique, in	111	29, 93, 94, 109, 112, 158, 205

(*Continued*)

(Continued)

Acronym	Full Name	Description	Page (Main Explanation)	Pages (Mentioned)
		which the knuckle is advanced until it spontaneously enters into the distal true lumen, which usually occurs in a very distal branch.		
Mini-STAR	Mini subintimal tracking and re-entry	Variation of the STAR technique in which a Fielder FC or XT wire is used to re-enter into the distal true lumen immediately after the occlusion rather than further down in the distal vessel.	111–112	93, 94, 109, 110, 208
Reverse CART	Reverse controlled antegrade and retrograde tracking and dissection	The opposite of the CART technique: a balloon is inflated over the antegrade guidewire creating a	133–135	45, 118, 121, 131, 132, 137,157, 202, 210, 244

(Continued)

(Continued)

Acronym	Full Name	Description	Page (Main Explanation)	Pages (Mentioned)
		space into which a retrograde guidewire is advanced—this is currently the most commonly used retrograde re-entry technique.		
STAR	Subintimal tracking and re-entry	The original antegrade dissection/re-entry technique described by Antonio Colombo—the subintimal space is crossed using a knuckled guidewire that is advanced as far distally as necessary to spontaneously re-enter into the distal true lumen.	93–94, 108	97, 110, 192, 208, 243
Stent reverse CART	Stent reverse controlled antegrade and	Variation of the reverse CART technique: a	134	131

(Continued)

Acronym	Full Name	Description	Page (Main Explanation)	Pages (Mentioned)
	retrograde tracking and dissection	stent is placed in the proximal true lumen into the subintimal space to facilitate retrograde wiring into the stent.		
Stick and Drive	Stick and drive	This is the standard technique for re-entering into the distal true lumen using the Stingray balloon. The Stingray guidewire is advanced without rotation through the side port of the Stingray balloon so as to puncture back into the true lumen. After confirmation of distal true lumen position with contralateral	104	

(Continued)

Acronym	Full Name	Description	Page (Main Explanation)	Pages (Mentioned)
Stick and Swap	Stick and swap	injection the Stingray guidewire is rotated 180° and advanced further down into the vessel. Technique for re-entry into the true lumen using the Stingray balloon: an initial puncture is performed using the Stingray wire to create a connection with the distal true lumen; the Stingray wire is removed and a Pilot 200 (or similar polymer-jacketed) guidewire is advanced through the same side port into the "tunnel" created by the Stingray wire to enter the	106	56

(Continued)

(Continued)

Acronym	Full Name	Description	Page (Main Explanation)	Pages (Mentioned)
		distal true lumen.		
STRAW	Subintimal transcatheter withdrawal technique	Aspiration of hematoma that develops during antegrade dissection/ re-entry crossing; can be performed either through the Stingray balloon itself or ideally through another microcatheter or over-the-wire balloon advanced next to the Stingray balloon.	107	108, 112, 209

Index

Printed in the United States
By Bookmasters